# Desperately
# Seeking Self

# Desperately Seeking Self

An
Inner
Guidebook
for
People
with
Eating
Problems

❧

*Viola Fodor*

**gürze books**

Published by: Gürze Books; PO Box 2238; Carlsbad, CA 92018; 760/434-7533

Cover design: Abacus Graphics, Oceanside, CA
Cover artwork *Women in Tight Spaces*, an etching by Sa Boothroyd.
Author photograph courtesy of Graham Paine, The Canadian Champion.

Grateful acknowledgment is made to the following for permission to reprint from their copyrighted materials:

Figures on pages 37 and 38 reprinted with permission from the copyright holder, The Creative Education Foundation, 1050 Union Road, Buffalo, NY 14224, from the *Creative Behavior Workbook* by Sidney J. Parnes.

*About School* from Jack Canfield and Harold C. Wells, *100 Ways to Enhance Self-Concept in the Classroom*. Copyright 1979 by Allyn and Bacon. Reprinted by permission.

Library of Congress CIP Data

Fodor, Viola, 1949—
    Desperately seeking self : a guidebook for people with eating problems / by Viola Fodor.
        p. cm.
    ISBN 0-936077-28-X (pbk. : alk. paper)
        1. Eating disorders–Popular works. 2. Eating disorders–Patients–Religious life. 3. Meditation–Therapeutic use.
I. Title.
RC552.E18F63    1997
616.85'26–dc21                                                97-16427
                                                                    CIP

First Edition

1 3 5 7 9 0 8 6 4 2

*This book is dedicated to all individuals
who are desperately seeking
to make sense of their eating behaviors
in the hope that somehow healing is possible.*

# Table of Contents

# Acknowledgments

In many ways, this page has been the most difficult one to write. I cannot begin to express my thanks and gratitude to everyone who has helped in the creation of this book.

Violet and Sajid Aziz, Sarah Mitchell, and Pamela Tames shared my vision. I could not have written *Desperately Seeking Self* without their encouragement and valuable editorial contributions.

Sa Boothroyd provided the riveting artwork for the cover. *Women in Tight Spaces* captures the torment, confusion, and helplessness experienced every day by those who struggle with eating disorders.

Wendy Barber, Bonnie Evoy, Noelle Ferraro, Kevin Fitzsimons, Erin Harvey, Janet Lovegrove, John Lynch, Christel O'Shea, Elaine Sigurdson, Anne Van Burek, and Julian Van Gorder read the manuscript in progress, helping to refine its message.

Frank and Violet Fodor, Elizabeth and John Hum, Tom Thomas, Sonia Kondrat, and Karen and Vernon Zelmer were among the other special people who believed in this project right from the beginning.

I'd especially like to thank my publishers, Lindsey Hall and Leigh Cohn, who love the book as much as I do and who have made a special place for it.

Many other wonderful people have contributed to this project in ways they may not even realize. They have enriched my life and supported me in my work. I hope that they know of my gratitude.

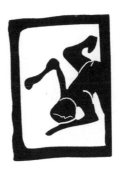

*If dis-ease is . . . a mirror of consciousness, then to fight dis-ease is to fight ourselves; to flee from dis-ease is to flee from ourselves; to succumb is to give up ourselves. The process of healing . . . begins not as a battle but as an opportunity to gain the awareness needed for physical, emotional, mental, and spiritual growth and integration.*

– Vivian King

# *Introduction*

*Desperately Seeking Self* is an invitation to healing—a passionate and compassionate call to you, if you seek freedom from your eating problem. If you are prepared to embark on a journey of self-discovery, it will help you begin to understand and experience the intricacies of self-healing in such a way that you can consciously apply them to your life on all levels. You will gain relief and freedom from your eating problem as you learn how to live more fully, with greater peace of mind and well-being.

I will introduce you to the healing process that has worked not only for me, but for countless people with whom I have worked over the past fifteen years. To help to make this content personally relevant to you, I have chosen a dialogue format to convey its essence— *a conversation with a woman who has bulimia*. The woman is a composite of my clients. In many ways, she resembles me many years ago!

You need not have bulimia to relate to this woman because she speaks in a way and describes a life experience that will resonate within, no matter what form your eating problem takes. If you struggle with compulsive eating, you will recognize yourself in her words even though you do not resort to purging. If you have anorexia, you can easily substitute "restricting," "starving," or "not eating" for many of her references to "eating" or "bingeing."

As you read *A Conversation*, you will discover that you have a great deal in common with others who struggle with a dark side of themselves and seek understanding and inner freedom. You will find reason to move beyond narrow definitions of who you are to one that encompasses your deepest level of being. Your true nature in its unadulterated form is the most precious resource that you have to help yourself.

There are ways in which you can become sensitive to this level in you. In particular, the daily practice of inner silence is a powerful way to nurture your true self and your full healing capacity. Because taking time out for yourself is so important, I have included a section called *Quiet Time* to help you to begin.

Although *Desperately Seeking Self* has few distinct divisions, you may require breaks. Take them when you need them or where they occur naturally for you. I would also like to recommend that you treat this book as a kind of healing reference to come back to again and again. You will find that as your awareness grows, you will read differently, understanding the subtle nuances of this process as never before.

The ideas presented here are not original. They arise from a perennial wisdom that transcends the ages and makes itself known in the lives of people who stop and listen to their hearts. Often, these inner truths surface when we least expect them—in our darkest hours, at a time when only spiritual comfort, guidance, and inspiration can have any meaning to us. If you embark on a journey inward, you will experience these truths for yourself. Even beyond that, as you find it within to stay true to your highest spiritual ideals, you will not only heal yourself, but find your place in the greater picture of humanity.

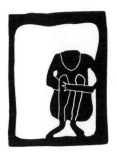

*I said to my soul be still and let the darkness come upon
me and know it is the Darkness of God.*

—— T. S. Eliot

# My Journey / Your Journey

## My Journey

For almost fifteen years I struggled with compulsive eating, fad dieting, anorexia, and bulimia—the full range of eating-related problems. This was at a time when eating disorders were closet behaviors. Consequently, I thought I was the only one in the world who relentlessly misused food and abused my body.

I developed eating problems easily enough. The erratic eating was there even as a child, but my body seemed to handle my poor choices. There appeared to be no consequences for my actions, so I did not care how I ate.

My carefree attitude changed when I turned sixteen. Somehow I gained twenty pounds and saw myself as fat. Convinced that I could never be happy until I was thin, I started to diet. Unfortunately, the more determined I was to stick to a food plan, the more my eating became unmanageable. Soon I became totally obsessed about food and my body, and my overeating spiraled into out-of-control bingeing.

In my mind, it was time to resort to more extreme measures. My new plan was to completely stay away from food. For months, I ate practically nothing and lost forty pounds. All of a sudden I was in fashion and I liked the "waif look!" But all too soon and without warning, my world came tumbling down when I could not keep up the restriction and the bingeing came back with a vengeance.

Devastated, but not prepared to give up the body that I had worked so hard to get, I felt driven to try even more desperate extremes. I somehow came up with the idea of throwing up my food. Although I found the behavior disgusting, I convinced myself that "the pluses" were worth the self-inflicted indignities. Now I had the body I wanted without struggling. I told myself that I would purge for only a short time, never thinking that I would not be able to stop.

Before I had the chance to catch my breath, my problem took on a wicked twist. True, I had the "perfect" body, but the purging behavior began to take its toll on a level that no one could see. Now, there were consequences to my actions. Self-hatred, guilt, shame, fear, frenzy, and madness grew with each purging episode.

Although I knew that I had to quit throwing up, I had now passed the point of no return. I could not stop, no matter how much I regretted my decision to start, no matter how much I prayed to come back to some sense of sanity.

The frightful realization that this behavior was out of control and taking over my life marked the beginning of more than a decade of hell. During this time I thought I was a crazy animal. I refused to seek professional counseling because I was certain that either I would be committed to a mental institution or put on display as a freak of nature for scientists around the world to study. Besides, I was too embarrassed to seek help. How could I begin to explain to a doctor that I engaged in this bizarre eating behavior every day and did not know how to stop?

I decided that I had only one option: to try to help myself. A logical step was to go to university to study nutrition. Perhaps if I knew more about how to eat sensibly, I could sort out my eating. I graduated with a Bachelor of Education in Home Economics, but *still* my eating was crazy.

Desperate and determined to get well, I enrolled in a postgraduate program, this time with a focus in psychology. Perhaps if I learned more about how my mind worked, I could help myself. I graduated with a Master of Education specializing in psychology and nutrition, but still my eating was crazy.

My eating and my life continued to get worse. By the fall of 1980, I reached my all-time low—I was mentally burned out and had no willpower left. I remember the day when I sat down in despair, resigning myself to the fact that I had lost the battle with this chaotic eating. I knew that soon the day would arrive when attendants in white coats would take me away because I was too depressed to get out of bed. Even worse, I might destroy myself with my insane and erratic behaviors. By this time, my bingeing and purging had become so violent that I was sure I would collapse in the kitchen or the bathroom during an eating episode. Or, if not at home, then on the highway—all alone, driving recklessly, bawling my eyes out while stuffing myself with chocolate bars and donuts. What disturbed me even more than my impending breakdown or death was knowing that soon everyone would see that I was not the perfect person I strived to be.

Resigning myself to this pitiful end, I finally let my mind rest. Besides, I was too mentally exhausted to think! But just when I thought that I had reached the end of my rope, with no reason to strive or fight anymore, a life-transforming experience occurred suddenly and unexpectedly. I get goose bumps even now when I recall it. Although I do not understand what it was, I do know that it gently and irrevocably changed my life.

It started with a feeling of being drawn to my living room window where I gazed out at the pouring rain for hours. I began to play peaceful music, the same songs over and over again. Somehow, spontaneously, I moved into a state of reflection—a different, quiet way of using my mind. Amazingly, that is when I began to change.

Over the next few months, as I spent time being quiet, my awareness opened and I started to gain insight into myself and my eating disorder. Intuitively, I came to the realization that *deep inside me was a core of goodness and value that was unshakable—even in the midst of an eating problem, even though my life was a mess.* I found immense relief and peace of mind in that. Knowing that I had nothing to lose, I took another crucial step: *I listened to and trusted in that inner dimension of myself.* Over a period of six to eight months, its steadfastness and wisdom gently guided me from the pit of despair to freedom and a new life.

In complete awe of these events, I felt compelled to sit and write about the transformation I had experienced. Logically, it was beyond my grasp, but insights were surfacing to help me understand its dynamics. It was as if the knowledge intrinsic to the healing process was now welling up, breaking through my conscious awareness. The ideas poured into words effortlessly. After several days, I collected my notes, exhausted but content that the burning desire to get it all down had run its course. As I examined and studied the ideas, I was truly amazed by their power and simplicity.

I was barely beginning to integrate the impact of this experience on my own life when another event took place. I invited a new friend to my home for dinner one night. Unbeknownst to me, she was suffering from bulimia. Arriving in a distraught state, Martha poured out her heart to me, as if sensing that I would be able to relate to her struggles from the depth of my being. She had been in therapy for years and was getting nowhere in her efforts to normalize her eating. I explained to her what I had been through myself and agreed to share with her what I had learned.

With trepidation and eagerness, Martha and I began an in-depth study of the healing process. We both wanted to know whether my learning experience could be helpful to her. In just a few months, as her awareness opened and she began to trust in the process, Martha broke through what seemed to be an impenetrable wall. She, too, discovered how to learn, to change, and to heal herself.

Before my own healing experience, I would have never considered guiding others through a process of personal growth. Although I had the academic credentials, I believed that I was too crazy to help anyone. But as I grew stronger, I began to see that I was developing a wealth of resources and knowledge related to the human capacity for self-realization and personal growth. Remarkably, the same force that guided me through my problems with food led me to my life work. Trusting in the inner wisdom that helped me to save my life, I opened my private counseling practice in 1981, the same year that I got well.

Today, this inner core guides me in every aspect of my life.

## Your Journey

*Desperately Seeking Self* is dedicated to helping you to connect with *your* core or true self so that you can listen to *your own* inner wisdom. My experience in working with clients has shown me that those people who get the most out of the healing process approach it in a certain way. Use these guidelines yourself:

## Open your mind.

Consider the possibility that this approach can work for you, that it may provide the missing link in your search for health and wholeness. This does not mean that you have to force yourself to believe in it or pretend that you do. Nor do you need to be overly zealous or gullible. Just see if you can suspend your resistance, judgment, cynicism, or doubt so that you can give it your full attention.

## Participate in this process.

Let yourself slow down mentally to experience what you are reading. You will derive no benefit by thumbing through quickly to gain an intellectual understanding of the content or by skimming through superficially, assuming that you have already heard it all before. If you truly had a grasp of these ideas, you would be living differently.

## Look to your self.

This book does not have the solutions to your problems—you do. At best, this book can guide you to explore a deeper dimension of yourself. If you can stop to listen to the silence within, you can begin to hear your own inner voice. It is the voice of healing, and it is as close to you as your own heartbeat, as your own breath, as your own prayers.

As your self-awareness grows, you will realize that your base of security is inside you, that your potential is boundless, and that healing options are open to you. You will find the courage to experience life fully, based on that deep awareness of yourself.

## Consider the questions that truly matter.

Some of the most important questions that you need to address are philosophical or spiritual ones. Your immediate concerns may center on questions such as these: "How can I get through the day? How can I stop all this craziness? How long can I keep fooling everyone?" If you pay close attention, however, you will notice that your search for answers penetrates a deeper realm.

Every day you are being challenged to make sense of a self-destructive impulse that arises from the darkest recesses of your being. Terrified and tormented by that negative force, you may feel compelled to question as never before the true purpose of your existence: "Was I put on this planet to be miserable? Is this what I have to look forward to until the end of my life? What have I done to deserve this? Who am I?"

Do not be fooled into believing that questions about meaning and purpose in life are too complex to consider or impossible to answer. If you attend to greater life questions by looking within, you will know how to answer them. You will be empowered to address your eating problems from a position of insight and strength.

## Start from where you are.

Inner growth is a process, a journey that has meaning and valuable learning each step along the way. Your greatest lessons are right before you. Once you know how to view your life experiences, you can begin to recognize the incredible learning potential in all of them—even in those that seem negative or empty. What you will discover is that even your fears and frustrations can serve the purpose of drawing your attention to deep, neglected issues and needs.

## Be prepared to be challenged.

You need to look at yourself and your life honestly, even if taking that step is difficult or frightening. As you acknowledge your real issues and explore them in a wider healing context, you will begin to see how you have been limiting yourself through your resistances, perceptions, thoughts, and behaviors. To carve out a meaningful life for yourself, you will need to challenge old ways that do not work.

## Be open to experience your pain.

Emotional pain has an important place in the healing process. You need to be willing to work with your pain, not deny or ignore it. There is no quick fix or instant relief—there is only learning through your pain and heeding the guidance of your inner wisdom. In her book, *Embarkations: A Guide to Dealing with Death and Parting*, psychotherapist Brenda Lukeman states,

> *"...if only we stop running, even for a little, we can see that the only true comfort will come from understanding, the only true healing will come from the truth. If we learn to listen closely, we will find that the pain itself has a meaning. It's there to be listened to."*

## Be patient with this process and with your progress.

You cannot deal with your pain or undo limiting and destructive patterns overnight. If you put external pressures or deadlines on yourself, you may slow the healing process or bring it to a complete halt.

## Accept the message in this book as a gift.

Bask often in its warmth and care. Trust that even when you feel immensely troubled, alone, and misunderstood, you can find the guidance and inspiration you need to be there for yourself.

Your attention has been drawn to this book because you are anxious to find relief from your problems with food. What you may not realize is that you have in front of you a unique opportunity to use these problems as a tool for self discovery and personal growth.

As you read the next section, *A Conversation,* use it as a resource to help you to open your mind to the basics that you need to explore for yourself on your own healing path. I wish you well on your personal journey.

———————— ✢✢✢ ————————

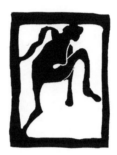

*...when the self has been confronted, when the hidden has been brought to the surface, the perhaps paradoxical result is not horror and paralysis—they come when the hidden has not yet been faced—but release and new birth.*

–A. J. Muste

# $\mathcal{A}$ Conversation

*For years I've been struggling with an eating problem. In the beginning, my bingeing and purging seemed to serve a purpose. I could eat whatever I wanted and still stay slim. Now this behavior has taken on frightening dimensions. My day consists of going crazy with food and trying so hard to stay sane. I hate being like this, but I don't see any way out. Still, something inside me won't let me give up. That is what brought me to you. I need help.*

It can't be easy to bare your soul, to be vulnerable, to trust in someone enough to share a dark part of you. Thank you for opening up to me. Please be assured that you have brought your concerns to a safe place.

You seem lost in your efforts to help yourself. You are wise not to try to deal with this problem alone. You need someone to assist you in the process of helping and healing yourself, someone who is skilled at the inner guiding process.

*What makes this problem so hard for me to figure out by myself? I'm bright. I try hard. I've read all kinds of self-help books.*

Let me respond to your question by sharing my experience. I struggled with bulimia for more than a decade. Each day I woke up determined to normalize my eating, once and for all. Each time I failed miserably. I did not realize that I had to learn more about *me* before I could help myself.

Remarkably, I came to some insights about my true nature before it was too late. Deep down, I began to sense that I had intrinsic value, that I had a wealth of inner resources, and that I could choose to be well. This self-knowledge came just in time for me to save my life.

*Your story is inspiring, but maybe you're special. I find it hard to believe that I can do what you've done.*

Don't lose sight of the fact that once I was where you are now. Perhaps I was even more downtrodden. Today I am well. My role as your counselor or guide is not to save or to fix you, but to help you to see that you are your greatest healing resource.

*All I need is will-power so that I can control what I eat.*

You are so caught up in your eating that you see it as the source of all your troubles in life. You see fixing it on your own terms as the cure, but your eating difficulties are only a manifestation of something much bigger.

Let me explain using the analogy of an iceberg:

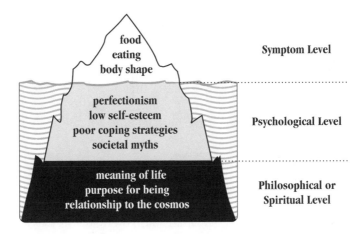

| | |
|---|---|
| food<br>eating<br>body shape | **Symptom Level** |
| perfectionism<br>low self-esteem<br>poor coping strategies<br>societal myths | **Psychological Level** |
| meaning of life<br>purpose for being<br>relationship to the cosmos | **Philosophical or<br>Spiritual Level** |

From your perspective now, you can see only the tip of the iceberg—the symptom level. Your real issues appear to be related to food, eating, and body shape.

But take a closer look. Just below the surface is another layer that represents the psychological level. This level relates to issues such as perfectionism, low self-esteem, poor coping strategies, and acceptance of societal myths that run contrary to your nature.

Now look at the layer that forms the base of the iceberg, and you will identify the philosophical or spiritual level. This level relates to your inner or spiritual self. It concerns issues such as the meaning of life, your purpose for being, and your relationship to the cosmos. The extent to which you attend to these core issues will determine how well you can deal with all of the others above.

Your challenge will be to open your mind so that you can consider the whole iceberg—all dimensions of your being. To heal yourself from your eating problem, you need to integrate your inner or spiritual self into your daily life.

*You talk about a deeper self. What if I don't have one?*

You have a deeper, spiritual self, you're just not aware of it now. Much like the part of the iceberg that is under water, you don't see it as real because it's beyond your range of perception. This simple fact explains why you can't turn your life around no matter how hard you try—*you are out of touch with the part of you that can help you.*

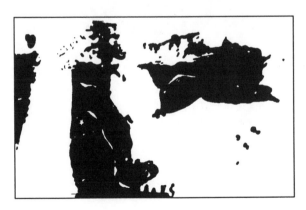

## The Importance of Perspective

It has been said that we tend to see things not as they are, but as we are. Indeed, we interpret life situations in ways that are uniquely our own. If our vision is muddled, if we view ourselves in narrow and negative ways, we cannot acknowledge the possibility that we have inherent goodness and worth or that healing options are open to us. What we don't realize is that *our way of seeing* is a big part of our *real* problem.

To help you understand the nature of perception and, further, the nature of self-deception, please take the time to do a simple exercise.

Look at the illustration below. Can you tell what it is?

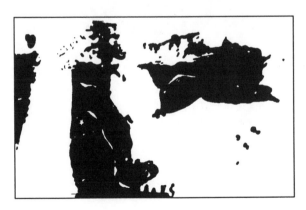

If this visual puzzle is new to you, recognizing its contents may present a challenge. All that you see may be a meaningless mass of black blotches on a white background. Try to identify it before you go on.

Now look at the next illustration. What do you see?

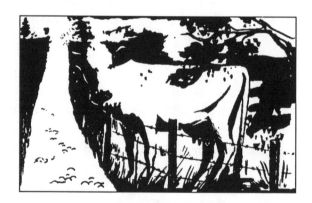

This illustration provides new information. If you look carefully, you will see that the image on the preceding page forms the head of the cow pictured here. In this puzzle, you can detect meaning in the midst of apparent chaos only by becoming aware of a more encompassing view.

We would like to think that reality is different from this, that we're too smart to be fooled. However, the same traps exist in real life. Even in our lives we don't always see the full picture. Unaware that we are deceiving ourselves, we still go on to make important decisions. These decisions will not be wise ones.

Simply stated, we must open our minds to these possibilities: *Reality is not always as it appears,* and *our present view of reality may not be our best option.*

*How does this relate to me?*

Let's take a closer look at your way of seeing yourself and your eating.

- You may be someone whose mood or sense of self-worth depends on a number on the bathroom scales. It won't matter how attractive or accomplished you are or how much life satisfaction is potentially available to you. That magic number will color everything. How can you view things so narrowly that you give those scales so much power?

- You may put blinders on whenever you binge. How can something like french fries and fried chicken become all-important? A one-track mind can lead to frenzied, inappropriate behavior. You might drive wildly to the nearest fast-food restaurant, stock up, and rush home. Crazed and in a trance, you stuff your face, all the while putting aside everything else—your commitments, loved ones, self-respect, true needs, financial considerations, and physical safety.

- You may be hooked on physical perfection, noticing every little flaw on your body, believing others like you only because of your looks. If you can't find a flaw at first glance, you won't let things be. You will use a more powerful magnifying glass to examine yourself. And because you believe so much is at stake, the slightest bulge or dimple, even if imagined, will become reason enough to lose five more pounds.

- You may base your self-worth on how tightly you keep your eating under control. How self-forgiving are you when you have eaten too much? You may consider eating that is not perfect as a cue to turn against yourself. You may believe that you deserve to be punished for being so disgusting, stupid, or weak.

If you recognize yourself in any of these descriptions, you have fallen into a narrow perspective trap. Distorted perspectives lead to inappropriate responses; they go together. That is the scary and dangerous part.

If you view yourself only in all-or-nothing terms or if you are filled with self-loathing, you may jump to conclusions or react impulsively. You may seek solutions in actions that invariably leave you more needy, damaged, depleted of resources, and out of touch with yourself.

*You're saying that I have to widen my perspective to make sense of my problem. That sounds fine in theory, but when I'm in the midst of a binge, all I see is food and all I feel is panic.*

When you are immersed in your binge eating, you may believe that it's impossible to shift gears or to act on your own behalf. Your crazy eating doesn't appear to be anything of your making. All you know is that you hate yourself for letting it happen, yet you can't stop it, and it's ruining your life.

This is an insidious form of self-deception. In your view, your eating is out of control and affecting every area of your life. In truth, you are letting food have power over you by not dealing with the real issues in your life.

*I'm helping myself the best that I can. Are you saying that I'm not?*

The survival instinct in us leads us to help ourselves in any way we know how, but at times we don't have the necessary tools to cope effectively. You may turn to food as an attempt to control many aspects of your life, not even realizing that you are doing it.

## Perspectives on Food

You may eat to comfort yourself, believing you need food to soothe you or to help you feel better. Do you binge when you are tired, bored, lonely, frustrated, angry, afraid, disappointed, or feeling fat? Food can be a powerful anesthetic to help numb emotions. People often eat instead of dealing with their true emotions. They confuse their real needs with a hunger for food.

You may eat to reward or punish yourself. Have there ever been times that you have dragged yourself home after a long and difficult day knowing that, no matter how bad things were, at least you could have something special to eat? Or have you ever managed to devour a whole cheesecake or a loaf of bread as a way to punish yourself because you didn't have the will-power to resist one piece?

You may see the shape of your body as your primary source of self-worth and personal fulfillment. In your opinion, the only way to create the physical image that you desire may be to ruthlessly restrict what you eat. Instead of respecting your true nutritional needs, you may desperately adhere to all kinds of unwritten rules for eating: "The more beautiful my body, the more valuable I am, so I'll eat like a bird to have a body that looks like a model's." Or, "those bumps on my hips and thighs make me look frumpy; I'll do anything to starve all those fat cells."

You may use your eating as a means of self-expression or as a way to define who you are. Fat can be a way of communicating, "Can't you see that I'm not worth knowing?" Someone with anorexia is often giving out a clear message, "I'm not ready to grow up or to be responsible." A woman with bulimia who flaunts her bikini-perfect body may be pleading, "I crave attention. Please give it to me. I need to be noticed to feel alive."

You may eat because you don't know how to just be. Perhaps, you don't know how to be with yourself in a quiet, nurturing way. Perhaps when you are alone, your dark side surfaces. Your inner demons come out. You may lose control and eat compulsively because no one is there outside you to keep those demons at bay. You may even be afraid to face yourself. Eating may be your only way of avoiding or easing the discomfort of being with that disturbing, confusing, or empty part of yourself.

Food can satisfy only one need—to nourish the body. You can't expect to get from it what it can't give you. You need to deal with your other needs and issues more appropriately. That is your deeper responsibility to yourself.

*How did my perspective get so distorted?*

You live in a society where it is easy to place a great deal of importance on external measures of success—often, physical appearance takes high priority. Many people use these external values to determine their priorities and goals. But that is not how life is meant to be, and you did not always believe this.

Consider this for a moment. Do you remember your life as a child? Was there ever a time when you were at peace with your body? A time when you ate in a totally relaxed and natural way? Could you eat when you were hungry, stop when you were full, and never think about food between meals? Do you remember a time when you experienced life in a more carefree, relaxed, exuberant, and balanced way? A time when your life experience wasn't constantly being interrupted by gnawing, obsessive thoughts of food, your physical appearance, or how you were measuring up?

*I do get a fleeting sense of such a time, but it seems like a lifetime ago. I remember the time I ate this incredibly juicy orange. I just wanted the taste to last forever because I knew I would be eating only one (it never occurred to me to eat more). I also remember the times my mother would have to shout for me to come in from play because my dinner was getting cold. I could eat and enjoy, but then I'd be on to something else. Eating sensibly was easy. Sure, I remember getting carried away with sweets and candy during holidays, and I loved special treats, but this food focus didn't go on every day of the year.*

*And I never used to despise my body when I was a kid. I just knew that this was the body I was in. It never occurred to me to compare my body with others and to dwell on my flaws. In fact, in my early years, I didn't even know how to compare myself to my peers! We were all equal in value, regardless of physical characteristics, family background, good or bad fortune, or idiosyncrasies.*

*I can't imagine ever feeling so free again. Sometimes I try to imagine what it was like. I even watch young children eating, hoping that I can somehow reconstruct what was there and get that innocence back. Sadly, it seems to be gone forever.*

Inner freedom is not out of your reach. You can begin to eat in a simple, natural way once again, treating food as food instead of loading it with emotional or symbolic meaning. You can become aware of your real needs on all levels and attend to them, rather than resort to excess, deprivation, or neglect. You can begin to see that your true identity and self-worth go incredibly deep; they do not hinge on your physical appearance or on your accomplishments. You can recapture a childlike wonder and be open to experiencing each moment fully, without any negative judgments or limited thinking getting in the way. Then, with this foundation in place, you can begin to integrate your new and evolving responsibilities with the experiences of adulthood to achieve a complete and rich life!

This is everyone's birthright. Yet, there are people who don't lead harmonious, fulfilling lives. Women, in particular, have come to believe that the more perfect their bodies, the greater the rewards in terms of social status, a better career, an ideal mate, happiness, a sense of value, and fulfillment. In their determined attempts to mold their bodies to some external standard, many get trapped in a vicious cycle of increasingly dangerous and desperate extremes. This cycle eventually becomes a way of life, further perpetuating the false belief that who you are is not good enough. It is how you look that counts.

*But it's true. Society does reward good looks.*

Yes, but what are the costs of these rewards? Will they bring the kind of fulfillment you desire? Is having the perfect body the only way to get what you want and need?

*This is really depressing. You are telling me that I value the wrong things. What if I don't want my values to change?*

You, too, have internalized the societal message that you are more worthwhile if you have a certain look. But are you ever satisfied with yourself? This kind of external focus can generate intense competition with yourself and with others. If you compare yourself to every other woman in the world, you will never feel slim enough, attractive enough, smart enough, fit enough, sexy enough, successful enough, or perfect enough. Any standards that you set for yourself won't be high enough when you meet them—you'll just raise them again. If you live your life by the rules of the perfectionist's game, you can never win.

## Changing Your Perspective

Something will always be missing as long as you ignore what you already know intuitively. If you are willing to learn how to listen to your inner voice, you will discover that you have value just for being you—a unique human being with vast potential and a purpose for being. You will begin to see your body for what it is—a precious gift that is in your care for as long as you are alive. You will want your life to be meaningful and balanced—a conscious expression of your true self. Your values will begin to shift naturally as you take the time to know your true self.

*I would rather try a route that doesn't require such close self-examination. It's second nature for me to count calories, plan meals, schedule exercise, measure my body, find gimmicks, and fake being together, but how do I*

*look into myself? I have tried self-development strategies before, but they've never helped. They mean nothing to me.*

Don't be so quick to abandon the process of personal growth because you have no positive experiences to report. Perhaps you haven't been ready for inner exploration. Perhaps the ideas weren't presented in a way that is right for you. If you close your mind, you can't begin to experience what this approach has to offer.

Your focus needs to change to a self-respecting, gentle, honest, internal one—your healing depends on it. As you nurture a relationship with your true self, your self-awareness will grow. You will discover your own inner truths. You will intuitively know that you can be well.

It is time to say "no" to surface solutions in favor of an approach that allows you to develop a natural, relaxed relationship with food and your body and that helps you to find peace within.

*That's great. I will get to really know myself, stop dieting and exercising, and turn into a blimp. I don't think you appreciate how important my appearance is to me.*

You've got the wrong impression! I'm not suggesting that you neglect your physical appearance. Nor am I underplaying the importance of fitness and healthful eating. These are vital aspects of a balanced life.

You don't need to throw away your rowing machine or your membership at the health club. Your body needs exercise, and learning about the nutritional value of foods can help you to eat sensibly. Just don't make these lifestyle considerations the focus of your life!

*Won't I get fat if I don't keep tight control?*

Rigid discipline that overrides your body's signals of hunger, pain, or exhaustion will not help to keep you in shape. The "no pain, no gain" mentality can only lead to problems and injuries.

Your body is capable of achieving a healthy and attractive weight, although it may not fit the perfect criteria of the bodies you see in glossy magazines. You possess body wisdom right now. Your body sends you loud and clear signals so that you can know what kind of care it needs. You are meant to be sensitive to when you are hungry, full, tired, stressed out, or pushing your physical limits. You likely repress or ignore these signals, listening instead to the thoughts in your head that tell you that you need to be paying attention to something else.

If you continue to ignore those signals, over time you can lose sensitivity to your physical needs. You can even grow to mistrust your body.

Many people believe that they can impose any demands on their bodies by restricting their eating, over-exercising, or driving themselves nonstop. Sometimes they push too hard, and the body rebels. They succumb to a binge, they injure themselves, or they crumple in exhaustion.

I am always amazed when clients arrive with extensive sports injuries such as shin splints and back problems. You would think that they were Olympic athletes training full time. I wonder how they have time to exercise so vigorously when frequently they are equally demanding of themselves in other areas of their lives.

The wear and tear is certainly there when people binge, vomit, use laxatives or starve themselves. How damaging must that be?

People can be oblivious to the detrimental effects of their behaviors, be it through unhealthy eating or exercise patterns, smoking, abuse of alcohol or medication, or lack of sleep. They torture their bodies, yet expect them to perform flawlessly. Some begin to believe that they don't care about any consequences.

*I am beginning to see that there is more to this problem than I had realized. I know my body can't take much more abuse. How can I begin to take that inner journey you describe?*

The process of self-healing will become real to you if you allow yourself to be sensitive to your inner world. For some people, that is a terrifying step to consider. In truth, it is scary only when you ignore it.

You need to open your mind to the possibility that you can face and be with your self directly. You are meant to be your own agent for healing and positive change. You can free your remarkable potential. Only you can decide how your inner journey unfolds.

*The prospect of facing and helping myself makes me feel overwhelmed and completely alone.*

It's okay to admit that you feel weak and vulnerable. After all, you are discovering that you play the central role in helping yourself, yet you feel totally inept. You feel stripped and stand naked, so to speak.

Ironically, this terror-filled time has a positive side. Because your old ways don't work, you are being forced to relinquish your false sense of control. In doing that, you are acknowledging that you need to refocus your attention and efforts.

Perhaps this gentle preamble can help you to open your mind—to truly "empty your cup"—so that you can begin to view your eating problem not primarily in terms of the hardship it has imposed on you, but in light of its tremendous potential for personal growth.

With the "untrained eye," you cannot see the healing potential in the challenges of your life, even though the opportunity is there to learn. If you are not sensitive to the inner realm of being, the purpose of your eating problem becomes lost. True learning stops and life looks overwhelming, chaotic, pointless, empty, beyond repair. When you know how to look at your eating in a healing light, true learning can begin. You will be drawn to your true life-path.

You are not alone in your need to explore this healing dimension. All individuals who struggle with eating concerns need to learn the same lessons as you. My own life-lessons finally became clear to me only after years of struggling to understand why I was in this frightful, insane situation.

## Life Stories

Let me introduce you to some people with whom you may have a lot in common. They are also at a point in their lives where they need to open themselves to healing options. While their names and some of the details of their lives have been changed, the essence of their life experiences still come through.

Joan came to me not through her own initiative, but because of her mother's prompting. Skeletal and blank in expression, she insisted that nothing was wrong and she could not understand what all the fuss was about. As far as she was concerned, it was her mother who had the problem.

David weighed two hundred and eighty pounds. He stood at five foot eight. He claimed that he didn't care about his size, but he was always careful to wear clothes that were so shapeless that they hid everything. His only friend was food. His main reason for living was to eat.

Marg knew that she didn't eat well. What woman did? What was wrong with throwing up every day if it kept her thin? In her view, she took care of herself. She was physically active, took vitamins, and kept some nutritious food down. Besides, her life was going her way. She was carefree and active. She could eat whatever she wanted. Life was so much easier since she didn't have to worry about every morsel of food that she put into her mouth.

Jodie lived in a lovely apartment by the water, but she may as well have been in jail. Nothing mattered since her dream of Olympic gold was shattered. Once the recipient of prestigious athletic awards, all she had now was her crazy eating. She hated being alone, but she couldn't bear to be with other people. She felt lonely, depressed, and inferior. One tormenting thought shaped her life: "I have failed in everyone's eyes." Collecting her antidepressants and putting them in a jar became one of her most meaningful daily activities. She vowed that one day she would take all of the pills and end everything.

Depression was Laura's middle name. For as long as she could remember, she'd had trouble with food. She had tried diet pills, diet foods, diet clubs, spas, antidepressants, megavitamins, hypnotherapists, and psychiatrists. Nothing could begin to lift her moods or tame her wild appetite. Laura had given up hope long ago. Secretive about her binge eating, she felt alienated and abnormal. When her husband was asleep or at work, her craziness would take over.

Jenny tried everything she could think of to normalize her eating. She even traveled to Europe and Asia hoping to escape her problem. When she returned, she realized that she had seen more bakeries and bathrooms than tourist attractions. Now she was into meditation and crystals. She was devoted to her high-power job. She had fancy clothes and a home furnished like *House and Garden*. Yet, no matter what she explored and accumulated, and what company she kept, nothing in her life truly changed. When she was alone, she would start to feel the deep ache, even in the middle of the night. She would find herself heading toward the kitchen to spend two or three hours satisfying what seemed to be a subhuman urge. Many of her female acquaintances envied her because she seemed to have it all, while her potential suitors found her unapproachable. No one knew of her personal struggle.

The bran, peanut butter, and honey combination didn't assuage Kim's raging hunger. The mashed tofu, wheatgerm, and banana didn't help much either. Bizarre combinations, she knew. But often that is all she would have in the house when she felt like bingeing. Funny thing, really. She knew so much about healthful eating—she even taught nutrition in school! Yet, she couldn't manage her own eating problem. Imagine the humiliation if her students discovered that frequently she would frantically devour all kinds of food supplies as soon as they left the classroom.

Heather's low self-esteem went back as far as she could remember. It cast a shadow on her entire life. Each success or accomplishment only made her more acutely aware of how unworthy and empty she felt. Her insecurities came through especially in relationships with men. No matter how much a man expressed his love and fidelity, she could not trust him. Before long, her mind would start to go wild with thoughts of his unfaithfulness. She constantly compared herself physically to other women, always magnifying her own flaws. Whenever her boyfriend was away, Heather would put her own life on hold, waiting for him to come back. Too upset to think clearly and too tired to resist, it would be at these weak moments that she would succumb to the secret urge that had become a big part of her life. She would raid her kitchen and tune out the whole world.

Claire was lost. She ate in a way that frightened her. She felt she was her worst enemy. Her parents loved and supported her, but their patience was wearing thin. She couldn't blame them if they gave up on her. Claire spent her life in the kitchen, the bathroom, and her bedroom. The laxatives were taking their toll. Twice she put off plans to resume university after having to drop out the first year. Any attempt to establish a normal life would collapse in a renewed effort to starve herself as soon as she stepped out of familiar surroundings. She was tired of caring. She did not know if she could go through the pain of trying and failing one more time.

Anne took pride in being a perfectionist. Everyone knew her as bright, pleasant, beautiful, and determined to get the most out of life. Always busy and involved, she did not seem to notice that her weight was dropping drastically. It was only when the panic attacks, fainting spells, and insomnia interrupted her schedule that she could acknowledge that something was seriously wrong. Anne was hospitalized for mental exhaustion. In a way, she was relieved to have some time out. Feeling lost, weak, confused, and disappointed in herself, deep down she dreaded the day when she would be back to all of her responsibilities.

Suzanne was in a good relationship, or so she thought, until the day her husband walked out.

After that, her life turned upside down. She couldn't begin to sort out her emotions. Intense emptiness, rejection, anxiety, and grief plagued her every waking hour. She feared having to stand on her own two feet, for they felt as if they were made of straw. Overwhelmed, she felt like hiding from the world. The only thing that kept Suzanne going was her precious infant son. She knew she had to take care of him, but she was terrified that she might destroy herself. Her long-time hidden bulimia was starting to rear its ugly head in a way she had never experienced before. Feeling desperate one day, she picked up her phone and dialed the number of a local mental health clinic.

Patrick's body ballooned over a period of five years. Each year he put on at least fifteen pounds. He gained weight not because he was oblivious to the problem. He was always dieting, but it never worked. For years he told people that he was fat because his metabolism was slow and because he came from a fat family. One day he came to the painful realization that the cause of his obesity was his overeating. Rather than retreat from this jolting and disquieting insight, he chose to become even more honest with himself.

Cheryl's purging started as an easy way to keep her body looking perfect so that she could feel good about herself. Many people found her gorgeous. Ironically, her looks meant nothing to her because of how she felt inside. She questioned her sanity whenever her eating got out of control. Her self-loathing and emotional pain became almost unbearable. As the years went by, her problem grew worse. While she became good at pretending she was happy, she sensed that unless she could calm the madness inside, her facade would soon crack. Driven to find a way out of the mess that she had created, she explored all kinds of alternatives.

For years, Sandy was unconcerned about what happened to her. Determined to jog along dark lanes at five o'clock every morning, she said she didn't care if she got mugged. Working seven days a week at two meaningless, high-pressure jobs, she rarely slept. A brush with death brought on by complications from starvation led her reluctantly to seek professional help. For the first time in ten years, Sandy was forced to slow down and face herself, a confrontation that she had been avoiding at all costs. Panic-stricken and furious because she could no longer follow her rigid routines, she believed that she would break down or go crazy before anyone could help her.

These are the troubled lives of people who experience eating problems. The Davids, the Claires, the Suzannes are unique individuals, but there is a common element among them. They have all known your kind of hell at some point in their lives. Take comfort. You are not alone, no matter how you feel. Others have been where you are now and have chosen to move on for good.

*It helps to know that I am not alone, but something worries me. Some of these people may get well, but I know that some won't, no matter how hard they try to help themselves. Do I have a choice?*

Unfortunately, there are people who will never experience true freedom from their eating disorders. Many do not have the opportunity to participate in personal growth work. Some do not care to, even when they have the opportunity. Some are prepared to settle for less than a life-enhancing solution. Some don't do well even when they put in the effort.

Without question, taking an inner route comes with its challenges. It is not for the closed-minded—people who already have their own agendas. It is not for the fainthearted—people who give up too easily or are unwilling to explore the unknown. It is not for game-players—people who will go to any extent to contrive strategies that have a payoff in order to avoid taking responsibility.

However, if you are prepared to learn about your true self and to take responsibility for your life, you will do well with this self-healing alternative. Only you can make the final decision whether or not to take this route. In this respect, you do stand alone. Your choice will affect the course of your life.

## Inner Work

*I am ready to work. I have nothing to lose.*

In making that decision, you are taking a crucial step in reclaiming your self and your life. The way to help yourself remains the same, no matter what has brought you to this point or how far you have plummeted into darkness. *You need to nurture your spirit and find a healthful balance in your life.* Inner work involves:

- claiming your true self and letting go of narrow definitions of who you are.

- opening your awareness.

- using your problem with food as a teacher or signal directing you to those areas of your life that require immediate attention.

- listening to your body's signals of hunger and satiation so that you can begin to respect your nutritional needs.

- embracing your full range of emotions and give them careful consideration.

- using negative experiences in your life as opportunities to become stronger, rather than using them to judge or give up on yourself.

- pausing throughout the day to release built-up tension.

- developing respect and trust for your inner voice, allowing it to guide you to a greater well-being and life purpose.

- quieting your mind daily to nurture your inner self so that you can access your full potential at all times.

- cultivating a deep trust in the healing process. Trust strengthens belief, and belief will open doors where previously there were only walls.

Over time, working on an inner level will allow you to know what you need and how to help yourself, not only with respect to your eating, but in every area of your life.

*There's so much to consider if I want to do this right.*

While you must be committed, be careful that you do not bring your perfectionism to your inner work. Healing is a process that you open up to, not an outcome that you can predetermine or control. True learning can't always be straightforward, pleasant, or easy. There will be blocks and setbacks.

If you can see difficult situations for what they are—life challenges—you can catch them in action and attend to them. It is important that you don't dwell on your weak areas. Recognize them, own them, and take responsibility for them. Do not punish or abandon yourself because you are the way you are.

Instead, extend compassion to yourself. Allow love and care for yourself to become the motivating forces in your life. While it's important to have positive expectations for yourself in every situation, you are setting yourself up for failure if you expect too much, if you can't let yourself be human. You will, at times, appear to be moving ahead at a snail's pace, but that is okay. At other times, you may think that you are losing ground. Even that is to be expected. As long as you are supporting yourself on the deepest level and are learning through your life experiences, you are still where you need to be: on-track and evolving!

To get well, you need to persevere! It has taken you a long time to dig yourself into a hole; you can't expect to climb out in a day. Your real test will be how well you can support yourself when you are down, not how easily you can coast along at times when everything seems okay. Your greatest learning may even come to you through your setbacks and most difficult times.

You are not alone in your need to learn more about

inner work. We all need to know how to be there for ourselves on the innermost level. An eating problem is only one of many signs that indicate a need to look within. Depression, panic attacks, burnout, drug or alcohol abuse, abusive relationships, identity crises, and lack of meaning in life are all signals to be heeded in a similar way.

*Looking at me, you'd never know that I had problems. I keep them so well hidden. Although I feel guilty, I have become good at leading a double life. There's the public "everything's-great" side and the private "I-can't-stand-myself-and-my-life" side.*

Many people lead double lives. They hide their dark sides and put on healthy fronts. Some people are so good at projecting a "together" image that you would never guess that they are struggling and tormented inside. They even fool themselves.

People with eating problems are everywhere. Their numbers are truly astounding. They teach nutrition, fitness, and stress management. They are in modeling, arts, drama, sports, and dance. They are in demanding business, academic, and health-related professions. They are at home, caring for others and maintaining households, often selflessly. They are young students on the threshold of adult lives. They are nurturing friends, life partners, family members, and contributors to society.

These are the same individuals who crawl into their homes when they feel overwhelmed. They pull down the window shades and unplug their phones. They indulge in their secret, shameful lives. Isolating themselves, shutting off meaningful interaction, putting their lives on hold, they do not emerge until the fear, pain, and frenzy subside. What is healthy and precious in each one of them becomes lost for a time to a side that seems wild, dangerous, untouchable, and dark.

*I feel trapped in this Jekyll/Hyde life and I hate it. You keep saying that I can be whole, that I can help myself far more, and that there is great learning potential in my problem. But right now I feel like Charlie Brown in that little cartoon where he says, "Life is full of choices, but you never get any!"*

I know that cartoon. Charlie Brown is making a snowball and his friend Lucy is approaching. She anticipates his next move. Calmly, she presents him with two options: he can either choose to throw or not throw the snowball at her. Further, she warns him that if he decides to throw it, she'll pound him into the ground. Not thrilled by the prospect of annihilation, Charlie Brown tosses the snowball away, drawing the conclusion: "Life is full of choices, but you never get any!"

Charlie Brown's words of wisdom might seem to fit his situation. However, they don't fit yours simply because the healing process is *self-initiated*. Nothing can keep you from taking full responsibility for your life, *if you so choose*. Even your problem with food can't stop you.

If you embark on the self-healing journey, it will unfold for you by itself. You can trust in that. Consider this one of the laws of the universe! You have the wonder of your true self to discover! You can learn of your power of choice. You can choose to be well.

*How can I be optimistic when I feel disgusting and out of control?*

You keep coming back to a common misconception— that you need to get rid of your eating problem before you can feel better about yourself and your options. I see things differently. In my view, *realizing your true value is a prerequisite for positive change.*

Our divergent perspectives in some ways remind me of the two opposing positions in the long-standing debate: "Which came first, the chicken or the egg?" In the end, it doesn't matter which came first, but it does matter how you view your eating problem. Your perspective—that is, what you believe to be true—dramatically affects the decisions you make and ultimately how your life unfolds.

If you are stuck in a self-defeating attitude, you will see no way to break free from your hellish life. Through your negative view, you will only perpetuate your life circumstances.

## Five Categories of Beliefs

Let us look more closely at the ways in which our perspectives shape our lives. Earlier I shared with you the life-stories of some people with eating disorders. Now we will revisit their lives to examine what they believe to be true. Because their vantage points vary, I have drawn up five different lists of beliefs to represent five categories.

Consider your life as you read through each list. Check off those beliefs that sound as if they could be yours. Be honest. Keep in mind, there can be plenty of overlap, so you may see yourself on more than one list.

## 1. Denial

In the *first category* are individuals who *do not admit that they have problems with food* even though they and others close to them may suffer the consequences. Denial is their distinguishing characteristic. Denial is the refusal to acknowledge that one has a problem and the need, if confronted, to disown it or blame someone else.

These are some typical beliefs associated with this category:

- I do not have a problem.

- If you think I have a problem, then you have a problem.

- Everything would be fine if my parents/spouse/ friends/co-workers/doctor got off my case.

- I do not want to change.

- I do not need to change.

- I know what I am doing.

- There is nothing wrong with me.

- I am in complete control of my life.

- If I can bring emotional pain to others for what they have done to me, there is a purpose in what I am doing.

- If I change, I will be like everyone else. Being like this is what makes me unique.

People who deal with their eating disorders in this way can't even start to work on real issues. Unwilling to budge from their "there's-nothing-to-take-responsibility-for" approach, they grow weaker over time. They don't let others in, and they don't allow themselves to reach out. While it can be painfully obvious that these people need guidance, they are quick to reject any assistance.

Let's reexamine the first three life-stories which fit into this category of denial.

Joan blamed her mother, so she was not open to any discussion. She ignored any indications that she had a problem: size six clothes that hung on her five-foot ten frame, raw carrots and clear broth at dinner for the fourth time that week, the friends that she shut out because she would rather stay at home in her room, the mother whose tears she could forget as soon as the pleading and fighting stopped, and the health professionals whom she methodically shunned no matter how hard they tried to help.

David couldn't see his problem either. He was happy eating man-sized pizzas or burgers and drinking beer. If other people did not like to look at him, that was their problem. His only satisfaction came from food and an easy, comfortable life—and he couldn't seem to get enough.

Marg needed her bulimia. She was a fitness instructor. A flat belly was essential, so she perfected her binge/purge regime. Marg could eat anything she wanted in any amount and still be in fantastic shape for class the next day. No one suspected that she had an eating disorder. In fact, she was a role model for many of her students. As far as she was concerned, as long as she could keep her tricks under cover, she was in control.

All these people refuse to acknowledge that they have any issues that demand their attention. Instead, they act as if they are fully in control, all the while entrenching themselves further in their destructive lifestyles.

*I can relate to this. When I had anorexia, I took pride in knowing that I was thin and bony. A good day for me*

*was not eating—I felt in control. I had all this energy and could go all day without taking a break. This was such a confirmation to me that my body didn't need food.*

*Even the bulimia seemed okay in the beginning. No matter how much I ate, I could throw it up. Soon I became trapped in that revolting behavior. Terrified, I watched my life spiral out of control. Now I hate the bulimia for what it has done to me and my life*

*Sadly, knowing I have a problem has done nothing to help me solve it. In some ways, it has made matters worse because I can see how helpless I am and how I am hurting myself. That only frightens me and makes me incredibly depressed. This nightmare with eating does not stop even when I desperately want to change.*

That is what most people with eating problems find out even if they felt in control of them in the beginning. No one who resorts to these extreme measures ever expects to get hurt or hooked. But even people who simply get caught up in perpetual dieting find that their lives can get out of control. Their worst fears are confirmed with each effort they make to resume normal eating.

## 2. Resignation

Some people even *resign themselves* to their situations. While they realize that something is seriously wrong, they feel helpless in trying to change it. Individuals with these characteristics fit into our *second category*. Consider some of their beliefs:

- I hate myself.
- I cannot trust my body.
- I am afraid of food.
- I am a victim of my eating problem.
- I am ugly.
- I am fat.
- I would rather be dead than fat.
- Life is not fair.
- I see no point in living.
- I am helpless.
- I am worthless.
- I can never be normal.
- Anything worthwhile is out of my reach.

- I see no point in trying to change. I have already ruined my life.

- The real world is far too overwhelming. I would rather hide, at any cost.

- I do not believe that anyone can help me.

- I cannot trust in anyone again. When I have in the past, I have been let down.

- I am not good enough to be close to people who are important to me.

- I would rather die than tell anyone what I am doing. I am so embarrassed.

- I do not know how much longer I can handle this pain.

- I am killing myself through this crazy behavior.

- I am an animal.

- I am losing my mind.

- I deserve to lead a miserable life.

- No one's life could be as insane as mine.

- At times, I wish I were dead.

These beliefs bring into clear focus the depth of anguish that some people experience every day. Their problems have become overwhelming and all-consuming. They feel it is pointless to put up a fight.

Remember Jodie and Laura?

Jodie's retirement from sports was more than she could handle. Just four years earlier, she was in training, her ambition set on being the world's fastest runner. When she didn't make the national team, she was devastated. She began deteriorating physically and emotionally to the point where she didn't have the energy to get out of bed except to scrounge around for something to eat. She felt that her life was over. She had nothing to show for her years of dedication and hard work.

Laura's depression affected all aspects of her life. She had already decided she would never have children. She could not bear the thought of not being able to bake cookies with them on a Saturday afternoon. And she would never want any child of hers to see the madwoman that she sometimes became in the kitchen. Besides, her future was just too precarious. She did not know how much more physical abuse her body could take or how much more mental torment she could stand.

*This is really scary. I share some of these beliefs. I see myself in these women.*

Even if your outlook is not as doomsday-black as this, it can still take its toll.

### 3. Ongoing Battle

In our *third category* are those people who don't completely give up; instead, they *wage an ongoing battle with themselves.* They may succeed for a time in fending off their inner demons, but, inevitably, their good intentions dissolve. They live in constant chaos and fear as they struggle to eat sensibly, only to fail miserably. These are some of their beliefs:

- Eating sensibly should be easy to do, but it isn't.

- I should be able to get my mind off food, but I can't.

- My life would be perfect if I were slim/if I did not have this problem.

- I will always have this love/hate relationship with food.

- I have to turn to food (or away from food) when I am upset or when things don't go my way.

- What I fear most in life is getting fat.

- I am afraid to be responsible—to stand on my own two feet—though I don't like being this way either.

- My metabolism has been ruined since I got into this. My body can't use food in a normal way.

- If I look at food, I get fat.

- It is my mother's/father's/spouse's/society's fault that I have a food problem. It has nothing to do with me.

- I can't be the person I want to be.

- What other people think of me is more important than what I think of myself.

- I can appear well adjusted and confident even if I am not. I can look happy or joke around.

- I cannot let anyone get close and see me as I really am.

- I want to get well, but I'm not prepared to ask for help. I need to get well on my own terms.

- My only hope lies in finding a magic cure or in getting some will-power that lasts. I have to keep searching until I find it.

- Someone else needs to fix this problem for me. I can't help myself.

- I shouldn't have this problem because my life has been good. I have great parents and a wonderful family. I have had so many opportunities.

- I am hurting people with my problem. I feel guilty about that, but I can't change, even for those I love.

- Until I get this problem out of the way, I can't get on with my life.

- I never thought that my life would get so out of control. I keep asking myself, "What have I done to deserve this?"

People who share these kinds of beliefs feel helpless in the presence of food most of the time. They lose sight of their worth, strengths, and potential.

Let's revisit a few more cases:

Jenny was living the single woman's dream, yet her life was hell. She was out of control. What better way to sabotage a lucrative career in sales than to miss making those important calls because she was too busy eating? Every time the pressures went up, her confidence went down, along with her ability to deal with most issues.

Kim's life wasn't much different. She wanted to eat normally, but couldn't. Anything over six hundred calories meant that she'd get fat. It's not that she was uninformed—she was an expert on nutrition and physiology. It's just that somehow her body was different. Whenever she ate more than she had planned, she would panic and binge. Then she would have to undo the binge. There was no way she could break this hellish cycle. While she maintained some semblance of normalcy to the outside world, she would be destroying herself when she was alone.

Heather's eating got worse whenever she was in a relationship. Every time her boyfriend so much as looked at another woman, she went into a tailspin, right in the direction of food and alcohol. Hard to believe, especially since she was talented, accomplished, attractive, and well liked by her friends and co-workers. Heather knew she had no reason to doubt her boyfriend, and she didn't like feeling jealous. Yet her insecurities would always get the better of her.

These people sabotaged the good in their lives and even harmed themselves because of the way they perceived themselves and their circumstances.

*I have felt out of control for years and although I fight it, I can't stop the way I think.*

Yes, you can. In time you can adopt a more nurturing way of being with yourself and shift your energies and resources away from destructive living.

### 4. Apparent Resolution or Recovery

At times, beliefs are not so obviously destructive. People in our *fourth category appear to have resolved their eating problems.* They seem to lead normal lives, but they still harbor considerable uneasiness and self-doubt. If they were to follow that gnawing sense that all is not well by being honest with themselves, they would discover that their lives are shaped by restrictions and boundaries like these:

- Eating sensibly is a constant challenge for me.

- I am okay as long as I keep busy.

- I am okay as long as I am not alone.

- I will never be able to listen to my hunger or trust my own judgment about food because my body doesn't send me any clear signals.

- I am okay as long as I stay away from certain foods.

- I can control but will never cure this illness.

- I am okay as long as I have ways to feel proud of myself.

- The pain of this problem will never go away even though I can move on to more normal living.

- I am okay as long as I can keep convincing myself that I am.

- I am okay as long as I do not look too closely at myself and my life.

- Although something is still wrong, I can pretend that everything is fine. I do not want anyone to worry about me.

- I am okay as long as I make money.

- Thank God I got rid of this hideous problem. Now I can be normal.

- I am okay as long as I have people in my life who love and support me.

- Although I have come a long way, this experience has left a mark on my life. I will always be damaged goods.

- For some reason, I was weaker and more vulnerable than other people, but now I have cleaned up my act.

Let's look at some people who share these beliefs:

Claire eventually managed to return to the university when she was able to put her anorexia behind her. She went into medicine, graduated at the top of her class, and became a dedicated family practitioner. By external standards, Claire had everything. But inside, that is not how she felt. She did not like herself. She would often get a sense that she needed something, but she could not pin down what that something was. Claire kept busy, hoping that activity would help dull the gnawing emptiness, but any relief was fleeting. She tossed aside all her yearnings for greater depth and meaning in life by deciding her expectations were idealistic. She concluded that peace of mind and fulfillment were only words. She would no longer look for them in her life.

Anne overcame her anorexia with the help of a local hospital program. She was adored by her husband and two children, was an exemplary wife, mother, friend, and community volunteer. Active, productive, and contributing to other people's lives, she was thankful to be free from her self-destructive behavior. Still, no matter how much she had to be grateful for and how much she gave to others, something inside her was dead. She thought that this was the price she would have to pay for what she'd been through with her illness.

Suzanne felt embarrassed by her past. She could still recall, all too vividly, the ugly food scenes and those years of hell. Her therapist reassured her that as long as she worked her twelve-step program, the compulsive eating would never come back. It didn't come back, but the chant, "once a bulimic, always a bulimic" echoed in her head. In some ways, she still saw herself as fragile. She was often on guard—to ward off what, she did not know. In spite of this, Suzanne experienced joyful moments. She was thrilled to watch her son grow up, and she was far more normal and healthy now than she could ever remember. She did not gain any weight when she quit purging, so even that longtime fear did not materialize. However, she could not understand how her life had come to this or why she still felt that she didn't know herself. Not getting any answers, she decided it wasn't worth her continuing analysis, and she quit trying to figure it out.

*If I could normalize my life to the degree you describe, I would stop complaining, too. Why do you find fault here? These women are now fully functioning. They're getting on with their lives and are healthy, productive people.*

Who determines the criteria by which to measure your life? How do you know when you are well enough or free enough from your eating problem? Do you view peace of mind and inner freedom as merely the "stuff" of wishful thinking or immature dreams?

We are all capable of personal fulfillment. People with eating problems are meant to learn from what they have experienced. Tell me honestly, don't Claire, Anne, and Suzanne seem scarred or boxed-in to you?

*What would you expect after all they've been through? Who am I to believe that I deserve more?*

It troubles me to consider how many people resign themselves to being less than whole, less than fully alive. Even you seem prepared to accept such a fate for yourself. This is a common view. It receives much outside support, even from some professionals in the eating disorders field who implicitly believe that people can never completely heal themselves from problems with food.

Please do not settle for a less than fulfilling life! If you accept a narrow belief system, you automatically limit your life because you can never imagine deserving more.

Our discussion of categories is not yet complete.

You have another category to explore before you draw any conclusions about where you belong.

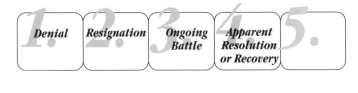

| Denial | Resignation | Ongoing Battle | Apparent Resolution or Recovery | 5. |

*What kinds of beliefs are left? What should I believe so that I won't limit my life and exclude the possibility of growth?*

Healthy, life-enhancing ones! You are now in direct contact with what is potentially one of the greatest learning experiences of your life. Don't waste it or throw it away. Your eating problem is attempting to guide you to wholeness. Use it well. There's no reason to settle for less.

Before I introduce you to the life-enhancing beliefs that the people in our *fifth category* share, I suggest you take a few moments to examine your life. You have spent a lot of time with your problem and you must have drawn some conclusions about your life and your self through the experience. What have you learned? Deep down, what do you believe to be true?

*I'm not ready to look closely at what I believe to be true. I have never thought much could come from looking more closely at what is inside my head. I've been looking for answers outside. This has caught me off-guard. You are asking me to expose myself to myself.*

I get this kind of reaction from numerous clients. No matter how many times I explain to them that they need to look within, they don't want to hear about it when the time comes to get to work. They don't think they are ready or strong enough to face themselves. Their fears and resistances are great.

Sometimes people say they want to be well, but they are prepared to get well only on their own terms. They say they want to change, but they are not willing to leave their security blankets, safety nets, or comfort zones. They would rather wait for the perfect time to start—a time when they won't be afraid or can be guaranteed that the outcome will be favorable.

*I am scared that what I'll find will be an exaggerated version of what I already see in myself when I am bingeing and out of control. I have put a lot of energy into hiding my dark side. What if looking into myself makes me more crazy?*

No wonder you fear looking deeper. You have drawn conclusions about your true nature based on how you have experienced yourself at the worst of times. Consider the tormented self-image that you have created. Do you ever see anything positive in yourself? Or is all that you see a reflection of your eating problem? If you removed it from your life, what would be left? Who would you be?

It is sad that so few of us can see our own goodness and true potential. All too often, we see our inner selves as the source of life's darkness, pain, and destruction. At best, you fear being disappointed upon looking within. At worst, you fear being destroyed. No matter how you look at it, you don't have any positive expectations about your inward journey.

Yet, this journey is a wondrous one! I chose to take it and I remember experiencing the same fears as you when I started. Believe me, there is nothing to fear by looking within, even when you find something you don't like. Whatever you learn will help you to free yourself from your eating problem. What matters most is the spirit in which you approach this challenge.

*I give you credit for being so optimistic! You obviously see more good in me than I see in myself.*

This is a good time for a story. Sometimes we can see important messages for ourselves through the lives of other people.

You have probably heard the story of Scrooge in Charles Dickens' *A Christmas Carol.* When I was a child, I dreaded the occasions when my family watched the movie on television. It was a sure way to dampen my Christmas. I would escape to the farthest corner of the house to hide from the haunting voices and chains, the eerie music, the anguished face of Scrooge, and the sad lives of the characters. But, I never managed to hide well enough. It was twenty years later that I could begin to appreciate the full meaning of *A Christmas Carol.* Now I love to use this story to talk about transformation.

Scrooge was just buzzing along in his life totally focused on what was important to him. His work was going well. He was making money, but he was a penny pincher. He couldn't understand why any of his employees should have lives outside of their work. He had no empathy for people who were less fortunate. He had no heartwarming traits at all.

Scrooge was not in the mood for company on Christmas Eve, but he had visitors anyway—the ghost of his deceased friend Marley, and three spirits that he had never met before. His life was the subject of their conversation.

The night to follow was long for Scrooge, partly because he was dragged through it three times, once with each of the spirits. Sparing nothing, they forced him to relive his Past, to scrutinize the Present, and to face the Future—the unknown. From beginning to end, his experience was a horrendous ordeal, filled with unwelcome self-examination and ominous foreshadowings. But the outcome—how can anyone forget the miraculous transformation? The miser discovered his heart of gold just in time to share in the true blessings and wonder of Christmas.

Scrooge found it remarkable that he survived at all, but he was truly awestruck by the effect that the experience had on him. He felt freed and exhilarated. He gained a new love and appreciation for life. He turned his focus and energy to living fully. Scrooge summed it up beautifully: "I don't deserve to feel so happy. I can't help it!"

Now, Scrooge wouldn't have changed if the spirit visitors hadn't arrived on the scene and made such a fuss. Likely he would have arrived to work even more grumpy than usual because it was Christmas. If the experience had not been so nightmarish, jarring, and intense,

Scrooge might have dismissed the haunting visions as a bad case of indigestion! As it stands, he was affected to the core of his being.

Scrooge witnessed firsthand the workings of the spiritual world. In that realm, anything becomes possible, any event can be orchestrated to benefit someone's soul. This was the gist of the spirits' message to Scrooge:

"Scrooge, you've managed to get off track. You've lost sight of the wonder of the world, of humanity, of yourself! That's not a good idea, especially since you were put on this planet for a purpose.

"You've become totally entrenched in a spiritless existence. That's not a way to live, but you don't seem to be able to figure that out for yourself. So we've come to help you out—to help you to see.

"We don't mean to give you a hard time, but if we don't, you'll miss the point of our visit. You are meant to lead an inspired life! Be sure that you learn this life-lesson now, before it's too late. If you do, you can become the person you were meant to be, and the pain of this nightmare will go away."

There are parallels in your life, although you may not see them. Just substitute Scrooge's obsessions with money and work with your obsessions with food, weight, and physical perfection. On the deepest level, you are not meant to—nor do you even want to—live a life based on those kinds of external priorities. But you have not known how to connect with a life that is more meaningful.

You don't have Scrooge's spirits to awaken you, but other events can serve the same purpose. Chaotic eating is a powerful teacher in its own right. It is no more mild-mannered or welcome, and no less terrifying. As distressing as it is, don't lose sight of why it is there.

*I find it hard to believe that something so terrible can contain anything good.*

I'm not surprised that you cannot grasp the true meaning behind your problem with food. Many of us don't know how to interpret philosophical or spiritual messages. We don't know how to learn from the dark side of ourselves. Instead, we do whatever we can to get away from it.

Don't run away from the dark side of yourself. Deep down, you already know that there is nowhere to hide. Now is the time to face yourself or your inner demons, so to speak. You can discover the gift in your eating problem. Therein lies the key to your freedom.

## Discovering Your Own Beliefs

Keeping this new life-direction in mind, let's come back to the task at hand. I want you to examine your own beliefs. Take the time now to write down some of your beliefs in the spaces provided on the following pages. Do not censor them. Express yourself frankly. Your responses may serve as a reminder of your progress months from now.

### MY BELIEFS ABOUT ME

I believe that I am . . .

**MY BELIEFS ABOUT MY BODY**

I believe that my body is . . .

**MY BELIEFS ABOUT MY EATING PROBLEM**

I believe that my eating problem is . . .

I believe that the cause of my eating problem is . . .

I believe that the way out of my eating problem is . . .

## MY BELIEFS ABOUT FOOD

I believe that food is . . .

## MY BELIEFS ABOUT MY LIFE

I believe that my life is . . .

*It is really depressing to see what I believe to be true, now that I am taking the time to be entirely honest with myself. I share so many of those destructive thoughts that you mentioned earlier— I'm afraid to let go of my eating problem because it's all that I know. I already feel that I've ruined my life. I don't expect to be able to help myself. I blame my past for bringing out the worst in me. No wonder I'm so miserable. I don't remember choosing to believe these things.*

I know you didn't willfully adopt any narrow, self-destructive beliefs. Still, as you can see, they are yours! These beliefs wield incredible power. They shape your entire life. You must challenge and discard some of them. Others you can transcend or outgrow. It will be up to you to establish a set of health-promoting beliefs or guidelines by which to live your life.

## 5. Healing or Transformation

All this discussion has been leading up to our *fifth and final category*. People in this group have recognized the learning potential in their eating disorders. They are *in touch with their true natures and are their own agents for healing and positive change.* See if you share any of their beliefs:

- My eating problem has been trying to tell me something all along. It is not bad.

- My eating makes total sense on this deeper level, although from my old perspective it made no sense at all.

- I can listen to my hunger, eat when I am hungry, stop when I am full, and enjoy what I eat.

- My life does not begin and end with being thin.

✳ • I don't need to have a food problem. Now that I have learned from it, I can let it go.

- I am not my body, but my body is mine. I respect and value it.

- I can deal with issues directly. I don't need to hide behind food.

- I can keep how I feel separate from how I eat.

- Life is rich, life is valuable, life is beautiful. My life has meaning right now.

- I have value being me.

- I am meant to be well.

- I need people in my life, but not in unhealthy ways.

- Balance is important.

- Solitude is the richness of self.

- Miracles happen.

- I trust in the process of life and in myself.

- I now know what it means to be patient and self-supporting. I accept that healing or getting well does not happen overnight.

- Setbacks are sources of valuable learning. Now that I know how to learn from them, I can use them to further my personal growth.

- My awareness is precious and important.

- My realm of responsibility extends to myself and beyond myself.

- I am contributing positively to the lives of the people I love.

- There is a way of life that suits me optimally, and I have connected with it.

- I love myself.

- I have forgiven myself.

- I have let go of my past.

- I do not need to be a victim of life circumstances, my family, my past, or society's values.

- I do not blame others for my problems.

- I have responsibility for myself, but I can turn to others for some of the resources and support that I need.

- I have given up my illusion of helplessness. I know that there are no limits to my inner resources. They will continue to unfold as I allow myself to draw on them.

- The whole point in working through a problem with food is to be free *from* something and to be free *for* something. I need to partake in life in a way that helps to enhance it for everyone.

Now we can fill in the final category:

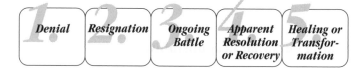

You can choose to be part of this fifth group that experiences a remarkable shift in perspective and new lease on life. All of these people have worked on their problems in a growth-oriented way.

*Aren't you being overly optimistic? Even so-called "normal" people don't think like this.*

I know your perspective is different, but this way of seeing is open to you. I have worked with hundreds of people who have experienced a lasting positive change in themselves because they have learned some fundamental life-lessons. Many of these people came from where you are now; they once shared your life-view and similar experiences.

To experience a shift in your thinking and to reap the far-reaching benefits, you need to participate in this learning process yourself. You get out of it what you put into it. That is the only catch!

## Taking Personal Responsibility

*Why is this kind of learning so difficult? I would rather read what I need in a book or get it from you than have to learn it for myself by going through it.*

You can't be involved in this process from the sidelines. Healing requires your full participation. So, I need to inform you that you can't learn on a meaningful level simply by reading a book. You can't get what you need through osmosis or by dependence on others. You can't fake, parrot, or cheat at this learning process. You can't buy what you need nicely packaged or in a pill, and you can't substitute something else to get the same result.

In short, there is no easy way, and no one else can take your trip for you. But that's what makes all of this so special when you do connect with it. The learning is so incredibly heartfelt and extraordinary that it will permeate every aspect of your life.

*You don't seem to understand. It's not that I don't want to help myself. I don't know how to do it.*

It is only a matter of time before self-responsibility finds its way into any discussions on healing. In a real way, you have created a block in your mind, one that keeps you from taking responsibility, one that perpetuates your learned helplessness.

You claim that you seek peace of mind, that you yearn to break free from your obsessions and fears, that you want to exorcise your inner demons. You say that you are willing to help yourself in any way that you can. However, is that truly the case, or are you caught up in wishful thinking or empty words? Are you truly prepared to do the necessary work or are you fooling yourself?

I have observed the phenomenon of learned helplessness in many of my clients. Even when they have the opportunity to get well, they shy away from the responsibility that accompanies it, sometimes not even realizing that they are doing so. Often they fool themselves into believing that they are helping themselves when they are merely going through the motions, engaging in intellectual exercises, grasping at short-term solutions, or feigning helplessness.

Many people do not realize how deep true self-responsibility goes. To be fully responsible for yourself, you need to listen to and honor your inner self. You need to be prepared to be your own person, to be accountable to your self, to be committed to leading an inspired life. People often resist taking this step because they are so far away from it that they don't know where to begin. Some people even abhor responsibility, seeing it as a burden, rather than the gift that it truly is.

No matter how you try to sidestep or avoid true responsibility, you will always come back to facing that same issue if you want to be well—there is no way around it. To experience inner freedom, to break free from your eating problem, you need to take full responsibility for your life. Inner freedom and responsibility go together. You will not find one without the other.

Only you can decide which path you will take, what you will allow into your life, how you will live every day. Only you can recognize your needs on all dimensions and be sure that they are nurtured. No one else can do that for you. No one, no pill, no outside event, no size or shape.

*It terrifies me to think that I will need to rely on myself. I don't know where to start. It seems to me that I can strive to be responsible to others, to my work, to almost anything else, but I don't know how to be there for myself— my mind doesn't work that way.*

I encourage you to give yourself permission to be a beginner in the personal growth process. Take the pressure off yourself. You don't need to come to this process with any great resources or tools. However, you do need to be willing to bring your true self, which will require a vulnerability, an openness, a willingness to being present in a new kind of way. It will mean allowing yourself to surrender to a greater healing force in your life. Your life-path will unfold naturally when you allow yourself to take that first step.

There will be a time that you will value true self-responsibility. You will feel fortunate to be in a position to choose what is right for you. You will have a sense of your personal power and find security in knowing that you can take care of yourself. No one or nothing can take that strength away from you. You can't follow in someone else's footsteps to get to your own place in the world. You have your own inner blueprint or map to honor, to use as your guide. No one knows better than you how you are meant to be living.

*I have nothing to lose by exploring this further. So, if I am willing to work on this, can I be a new person? Will my eating problem go away?*

You appear to be ready to take on the challenge of being responsible for your self, but here's a word of caution. At first glance you might think that all that's required of you is to make up your mind to be optimistic. But it will not be enough. Trying to convince yourself to be positive is commendable, but it's not genuine. At times, positive thinking is little more than positive reprogramming—just another external and artificial way of shaping ourselves.

Nor can you simply make up your mind to follow a positive plan of action and use will-power to follow through. You will fall short of your goals using such an approach, no matter how committed you are.

## Discovering the Inner Self

*Well, if I can't talk myself into being healthy-minded or force myself to be different, what else can I possibly do?*

Using your logical thinking and will-power in a more spiritually sensitive way will not help you to find your true life-path. Instead, I would suggest that you take time out to explore the deeper realm of self directly, experientially. Then, you can come to these realizations:

Your inner self is real. It is part of a spiritual dimension. You are meant to awaken to your true self and to bring it into your daily life. When you connect with your true self, you will know that you have value and that you are here for a reason. Given time, the inner self will become more real to you than anything else in your life.

You inner self is wise and strong. You have an abundance of inner resources on which to draw. Your healing potential is boundless. Deep down, you already know what you need and how you are meant to be living.

Your inner self is always there to help you. Your inner self is forever present. It can help you through any life situation. If you are prepared to listen to your inner voice, you will receive guidance and support whenever you need it.

The healing process is innate. The healing process exists within you, but it also extends beyond you because it is part of a greater benevolent force. Consequently, you don't need to make healing happen in your own limited ways. Instead, you need to create the right conditions so that it can unfold in your life. Healing happens by itself when you open up to it.

As you discover these truths, you will know that you are your greatest resource. You have had it inside you all along.

*This self-help approach puts responsibility into a new light for me. I can't believe that I am considering it.*

Without question, this approach requires a new kind of commitment and a leap of faith! You will be stepping into the unknown and building a life, all the while depending on yourself in a way that you have never dared to before.

## Quieting the Mind

Let's start with the basics of this process. As a first step, in order to establish a relationship with your true self and to evoke your full healing capacity, you will need to learn to be with yourself in a calm, receptive, reflective way. Be prepared to learn how to quiet your mind! In complete inner silence, many of life's secrets can be revealed to you.

*My mind is always going. I can't turn it off. Sometimes I can't even sleep. Even when I am not immersed in crazy eating, I am still engaged in crazy thinking!*

Many of us have fallen into the active mind trap. Even if we are free from debilitating obsessions or worries, we're still in a constant whirlwind of mental activity—planning, researching, analyzing, organizing, studying, resolving, rehashing, rehearsing, refining, remembering, regretting, juggling, drifting, fantasizing, or playing mind games.

Much of this inner chatter is excessive or useless, even damaging. But we do have a choice—we can turn it off.

To transcend your perceived limitations, to develop your highest potential, to connect with a spiritual sense, you will need to learn how to reflect. In quieting your mind, you move from an active into a receptive state of mind. You are no longer locked into your old perspective, one shaped by your usual, constant thinking. You will be free to explore who you are and what reality is all about from an inner point of view.

When you bring a quiet mind into your daily life, personal growth takes on an entirely new dimension, one characterized by a deep and profound clarity and personal fit. Words such as wisdom and inner strength will no longer be empty to you. They will come alive—you will experience them.

*So if I learn how to quiet my mind, I can free my potential?*

That is right. However, I'm not implying that simply quieting your mind will resolve all your problems. Quieting your mind will give you access to an inner reservoir of resources, but you still need to support yourself. You still need to apply your newly-developing abilities consciously and deliberately until they come naturally to you. This is part of your inner work.

It will be worth the effort. You will move into a new realm of possibilities, one that would not otherwise be open to you. The path to discovering your self and realizing your potential is the same one you must take to heal yourself from an eating problem.

*I would love to live that way. Tell me more. I am starting to look forward to all of this.*

It is refreshing to hear you speak with inquisitiveness and enthusiasm. You have every reason to feel inspired by the benefits that you will experience if you make personal growth a priority. Let me expand on some of them.

### The Benefits of Inner Work

When you learn how to reflect, your awareness opens, and you can put things in perspective. You can move beyond confusion and chaos to seeing a meaningful whole. You will see your problems with food in the context of your entire life. With clear vision, you can begin to identify the issues that you need to address and understand how to work on them.

Important issues will come spontaneously into your conscious awareness. You do not have to actively seek them out. It will be apparent which ones take priority. While at first you may be alarmed or caught off-guard by your penetrating insight and wisdom, in time you will value the direct route that you have to your innermost self.

When you know how to reflect, you can begin to answer questions such as these: "Who am I? Why am I here? What is life all about?" These questions relate to issues with which we all struggle. You need insight into your true nature if you are to help yourself. How can you know your needs and true potential when you don't even know who you are?

We hunger for philosophical learning but have few opportunities to explore our true natures in any authentic way. We have never learned that when we are with ourselves quietly, in inner silence, we can find meaningful answers to fundamental questions. We can begin to hear the voice of wisdom within.

When you know how to reflect, you can step back from your life concerns, viewing them from the vantage point of your inner self. You can address all your life issues from the center of your being in a calm, objective, creative, and powerful way.

When you can sit with a quiet mind, you will find that you can deal with even the most disturbing issues and feelings without becoming overwhelmed by them. You will no longer feel compelled to turn to food as a way to escape or to cushion your discomfort and pain. You

can work through even your most confusing and agonizing feelings, healing yourself emotionally.

You will find new meaning in your emotional pain.
You will discover that suffering is not the unfortunate
outcome of life's trials or a state in which to dwell forever. Nor is it a confirmation that you are useless or that
life is pointless and unfair. Rather, it serves the purpose
of drawing your attention, directly and forcefully, to
your life lessons. If you are willing to give your painful
emotions the attention and care that they need, they
will carry you to greater levels of spiritual insight and
inner freedom.

Even the challenge of coming to terms with your past
will be one that you can take on with equanimity and
grace. You will benefit from viewing your past gently
and compassionately in light of your expanded awareness. You will find this approach more productive than
reliving each painful incident, delving intrusively, or
laying blame.

Quieting your mind plays a key role in enhancing body
awareness. When your mind is still, you can turn your
full attention to being in touch with your body. Rather
than listening to that misinformed "tape" in your head—
the one that seems to know all the answers—you can
tune in to your body, thereby establishing a clear, direct, accurate communication link. You can begin to

develop a sensitivity to your body's true signals related to hunger, satiation, built-up tension, physical exhaustion, and mental fatigue.

Quieting your mind, then, will allow you to identify real needs and issues and to attend to them in a way that is immediate and direct. This increased awareness and ability to act on your own behalf will empower you as never before.

## Will vs. Will-Power

*I can see it's time to let go of my long-held belief that logic and will-power are my most valuable self-help tools.*

This is a realization that we all need to come to before we can help ourselves. For years, I looked for a cause for my eating problem, a logical solution, a reason for my insanity. Unfortunately, I was attempting to find answers to a problem that I had not yet clearly identified, and one for which there were no logical answers. After years of searching, I had more questions than answers and felt more defeated than ever. I concluded that something was drastically wrong with me and that my problem was insurmountable. I was wrong on both counts.

Now I know differently. Now I can see how our problems can become larger than life if we do not have the inner tools and resources to deal with them. It is not so much the problems themselves that defeat us, but our ways of working with them. We owe it to ourselves to discover our capacity for helping and healing ourselves. That will mean moving beyond our reliance on logical thinking and will-power as our greatest self-help tools.

Logic is certainly a powerful and essential tool, but applied to certain life challenges, it is useless. For these kinds of problems—and an eating disorder falls into this category—we need another way of using our minds, and that is to suspend our logic and move into a state of reflection. This is when our thinking becomes creative, healing, and wise.

Will-power will also bring disappointing results. When we experience the natural, and often effortless, strength of will (as opposed to will-power), it becomes apparent how forced, limiting, and exhausting will-power is.

To help you understand the subtle, yet significant difference between will and will-power, I would like to recount a little story entitled, *The Animal School.* You will find the complete story in Leo Buscaglia's book, *Love.*

One day some animals got together in the forest with the intention of starting a school. There was a rabbit, a squirrel, a bird, a fish, and an eel. In selecting the core or compulsory subjects, the animals considered each other's special talents. They believed that they would all benefit from learning what each animal did best. Problems started immediately.

Because the squirrel excelled in perpendicular tree-climbing, it was included in the curriculum. But, when the rabbit started his tree-climbing course, he didn't do so well. He kept falling over backwards and landing on his head. Before long, he developed terrible headaches. He could no longer run, an activity in which he had always excelled. And no matter how hard he tried, he couldn't climb trees!

The bird did wonderfully in flying, but he ran into serious problems when he started burrowing into the ground—he kept breaking his beak and wings! Soon he was making a C in flying and an F in burrowing, and he had a hellava time with tree-climbing. The story continues with the ill-fated attempts of the other ambitious animal students.

Just consider the rabbit's folly. He was attempting to climb a tree—an impossible feat. Imagine the kind of effort he must have expended. Is it any wonder that he fell and landed on his head? The bird didn't do any better in his attempts to dig holes. He realized too late, after he seriously injured himself, that his body wasn't designed for that activity.

It would be easy to laugh at these animals for their foolishness. But as human beings, many of us get equally out of touch with what truly works for us or how we are meant to be living. Many of us live our lives by unwritten rules that prevent us from becoming our unique selves.

Sometimes we mistakenly believe that we can force ourselves to do anything. In our overzealous efforts to meet certain standards or to accomplish our goals, we resort to will-power. The price we pay for the obsessive, blind effort is high: we weaken, numb, hurt, or destroy ourselves. Alternatively, we may decide we are failures and give up altogether when we don't get the results that we want.

Just consider the different outcome if the rabbit had stopped for a moment to check in with his instincts or his inner sense of what works for him as a rabbit. What if he had realized, "Hey, I am a rabbit! I don't belong in any tree!" If he had been in touch with his true nature (perhaps by taking a basic course in "How to Be True to Your Self"), he would have known enough to stay out of trees. He wouldn't have considered climbing one. In fact, his will wouldn't have let him.

This brings us to the subtle distinction between will and will-power. Will is naturally protective. We can only use will according to our true natures, not against them. The more we have a true sense of ourselves, the more difficult it is to become trapped in any kinds of patterns or situations that aren't good for us. We are naturally drawn toward experiences that allow us to care for ourselves and to actualize our unique potential.

See the difference? The kind of strength so many people use is the uninformed, crude, surface effort of will-power. Will, or true inner strength, comes from a deeper, wiser, life-enriching source.

Knowing that this difference exists between will and will-power is crucial to your full understanding of where your strength comes from to help you deal with your eating problem. The way to break free is not to use will-power to force yourself to change. Instead, you need to develop and nurture your inner self, so that you can access your will. In other words, the wisdom and strength that come from realizing your true self are the resources you need to liberate yourself from your destructive eating behaviors. Deep down, you too, have an instinct, an intuition of what is right for you—no matter how far removed you have become from that wisdom.

As a matter of interest, the eel in this story became the class valedictorian! Like the other animals, he wasn't in touch with his true nature, nor was he leading an especially fulfilling life. He simply plodded along, without making any effort. However, the eel's saving grace was that he didn't burn out or maim or injure himself as did the others because he didn't even try!

*I can relate to the rabbit. I may not be climbing trees, but I feel as if I am spinning my wheels or beating my head against a wall. It's a chore just to get through the day. It looks as if part of my problem is that I'm thinking too much and trying too hard. That is all I know how to do. As I have never experienced a deep sense of myself, I'm still not sure what I am looking for. What exactly is the self, and how can it be so important?*

Your life is not meant to be as difficult as you have made it. Your life can begin to flow.

## The Inner Self

You have within you an essence, a core, your essential self. It goes deeper than all of your limiting, negative self-identities. You may see yourself primarily as *a failure, a body, a fat body, a walking eating disorder, a victim, a phony, an impostor, a crazy person, a nobody, damaged goods, or a lost soul.* Yet, you are none of these. Nor are you any of the other careless or demeaning labels that you have pinned on yourself in ignorance of your true nature.

People experience self in different ways. Some describe it as an *inner light, Higher Self, the Source, Consciousness, Spirit, as God-like, inner calmness, or awareness.* As one of my clients announced with absolute joy, "There is a *me* in there that is connected to finer and greater things!"

When you experience self, you know it. Every situation, every aspect of your life will be suffused with awareness, beauty, compassion, goodness, wisdom, and strength. It is only when you are not connected to your inner self that life can seem shallow and pointless, even desperately out of control.

Let me tell you Megan's story. I still remember the first time Megan came to see me. At twenty-three years of age, she had already experienced enough anguish and disappointment to last an entire lifetime. Painfully and in a whisper, she related to me the trials of the previous six years—the terrifying love/hate relationships with abusive men; the bitter disputes with her family and their rejection of her; her series of dead-end jobs and her failed efforts to secure meaningful work; her vaga-

bond existence perpetuated by her running away, trying to find herself; the black hole of depression she
experienced all too often; the memories of her youth
that still haunted her; her financial burdens; her abor-
tive efforts to find professional counseling; the devastating losses and disappointments generated, in part,
by her negative emotions and erratic behavior; her fear
of intimacy and her inability to trust; and the daily
bouts of crazy eating, sometimes accompanied by alcohol abuse.

Megan had lost her capacity to feel positive emotions
such as love, joy, appreciation, and playfulness. She
was afraid that she was forever scarred so that even if
her bulimia went away and the severe depression lifted,
her life would not be worth living.

While there was little I could do to bring Megan instant relief, I shared my observations and hopes with
her. I wanted Megan to see that her present situation
was not meant to signal the end of her life, but to usher
in a new way of living. If she could let herself learn
from her circumstances, no matter how desperate they
might seem, she could transform her life.

I want to convey the same basic message to you. You
are unique and so is your situation. Still, on a fundamental level, your concerns and life-lessons are universal. *The most significant challenge in life for you, as it is*

*for each of us, is to find your way back to your inner or spiritual source.*

Because Megan was so distressed, I used much of our time together introducing her to the exercise that I call *Quiet Time.* I wanted her to know that she could connect with her spiritual self and initiate the self-healing process if she could learn how to quiet her mind.

Megan was surprised to hear that Quiet Time could be so important. As a child and young teenager, she had frequently spent time in simple activities that allowed her to be alone and quiet. Not realizing the value of this time and being encouraged by others to use it differently, she had let it slip away.

Megan promised that she would try Quiet Time that very evening. Because she felt fragile and vulnerable, we parted, agreeing to meet the following day.

When Megan came in the next morning, there was a sparkle in her eyes. The tension was gone from her face. It was as if a great burden had been lifted from her shoulders. Megan told me how, to her amazement, she could get into Quiet Time. Even more incredible to her were the insights she had as she sat there, calm and at peace with herself.

For those few peaceful moments, troubles and traumatic events could not touch her—she was separate from them! Deep inside, she did not feel scarred. Then this idea occurred to her: if she could strengthen the connection to this untouched core and take it into her daily living, in time she would have the substance and strength to break free from the negative influences that had held her captive for so many years. In essence, she would be free to begin a new life. Generally, such insights do not come so quickly for my clients. For Megan, they could not have come at a better time.

*I want to be strong. I want this inner freedom that you are talking about. How can I learn how to quiet my mind and get to know my self?*

You will find what you need in the basic exercise Quiet Time. Simply stated, what I want you to do is to spend a minimum of fifteen minutes a day sitting still and doing nothing.

*How could I ever sit still and do nothing? I deliberately try to keep myself busy so I won't get depressed or feel afraid. And keeping busy helps me to avoid food.*

While it will be a challenging task, you can learn how to quiet your mind. You were born with this capacity.

But in the process of growing up, you failed to develop it. We live in a society that values the abilities to reason and analyze. Not recognizing the importance of reflection and intuition, most of us abandoned these essential mind functions early in our lives.

In essence, what you are doing in Quiet Time is taking the opportunity to learn how to use your mind fully and freely. You are giving yourself space to begin to relate to yourself in a nourishing way that goes beyond active, conditioned thought.

### The Essence of Quiet Time

Let me draw your attention to the key elements of Quiet Time. During Quiet Time, you take time to be alone with yourself. Give yourself permission to set aside everything you would normally be thinking about—your roles, responsibilities, relationships, problems, worries, regrets, circumstances, plans, fantasies—to be in your own quiet company. Choose a setting that is free from external distractions. Unplug the phone, turn off the radio, and find a comfortable chair.

Cultivate a suitable inner environment as well. As a first step, you may find it helpful to bring your attention to your breathing. As your breath rises and falls, commit yourself to sitting in silence. Once you are quiet, bring your attention to your thinking. Now, begin to observe your thoughts with the intention of letting them go. In a way, you are emptying your mind. As you sit comfortably and a thought comes to mind (perhaps related to a person who is important to you), acknowledge the thought and gently usher it out of your mind. While the thought may be important, you can come back to it later. Your immediate task is to quiet your mind. Then, as other thoughts surface (perhaps related to your eating), repeat the letting-go process.

What do you think will happen the first time you take Quiet Time?

*There's no way it will work. I'll be bombarded with thoughts of all kinds. My mind will be racing—regretting that I ate so much junk food last night, regretting that I ate anything at all, endlessly counting calories or fat grams, tormenting myself about how terrible I look or how useless I am, wondering why I am so screwed up, being hard on myself because this Quiet Time isn't working, and agonizing over that ever-present concern: "How am I ever going to solve this terrible food problem?"*

You are describing the kind of active mind resistance that most people experience in their early attempts to take Quiet Time. Even people who like to think of themselves as free thinkers realize through an exercise like this that they are free thinkers only to a point. Beyond that point, something automatic clicks in.

When people find it impossible to relate to Quiet Time, they want to quit. They conclude, "This is too hard. I can't be bothered. I'll come back to it later when I'm more in the mood or when I have more energy or time." Some people become incredibly creative in finding reasons for not taking Quiet Time.

If you experience this, please don't become so discouraged that you let yourself give up. Instead of seeing your mind's resistance as a reason to quit, you need to see it as a reason for concern. Your mind's unwillingness to slow down is only a sign of how much your thinking is out of control. As long as your thinking is out of control, you can't help yourself.

Fortunately, your mind will start to co-operate if you continue your daily practice. It will slow down because you are training it to do so. Mind-training is an important tool that ultimately gives you the freedom to let go of unwanted thoughts and to replace them with self-supporting ones. In a direct and practical way, this mind tool will help to strengthen your will, that ability to follow through on your innermost wishes and desires.

*You can't imagine how free I would feel if I could choose my own thoughts and follow through on my good intentions. So do you think that one day I can have a healthy relationship with food, rather than succumb to all the usual temptations?*

The ability to choose what is right for you may come sooner than you think. Let me give you a practical example of how this works. Let us say that your favorite dessert is in the fridge. You know it's there, and you can't stop thinking about it. It seems as though the black forest cake or white chocolate mousse is calling to you. While your body knows that it does not need more food, your mind has different plans for you. It is tyrannizing you with statements like, "You have to eat some. You can't just leave it there. Think about how much better you will feel when you eat it."

Those old rationalizations seem to surface from nowhere, and you don't have the strength to intercept them. Something outside the rational, sensible you is irresistibly aroused. Won't it be an accomplishment when you can say to yourself, "I don't need any dessert; I will go and read my book instead," and be able to follow through?

Here is another example of the difference getting your thoughts under control can make in your life. Let us say that you have spent the day with friends. They are now ready for dinner; you are ready for your aerobics class. On one hand, you resent their wanting to eat, thereby putting a damper on an otherwise good day, yet you are upset with yourself because you can't be flexible and "normal." You decide to be social, but even before your group arrives at the restaurant, your mind is grinding out of control. There are two voices at war in your head. Once takes this position, "I'll eat something small. Tomorrow I'll starve and exercise two extra hours." The other voice rebels, "Are you crazy? This food is loaded with fat. Eat and you'll blow up like a balloon overnight." It doesn't matter which voice you listen to because neither one allows you to take care of yourself— you lose either way.

Won't it be freeing when, instead, you can give yourself permission to eat, enjoy the meal and the company, have a fabulous time, and wake up the next morning ready to begin a new day?

Helping yourself is a matter of being able to pause long enough to realize that your rationalizations are just lame excuses. When you pause and center in yourself, you can become aware of what you need to be doing in the present moment. You can draw on your intrinsic strength to challenge old thoughts and to select a new option.

You need to be in control of your thinking before you can hone this essential skill. You are meant to have the freedom to choose your own responses to life events, rather than be a victim of food, your body, habits, impulses, cravings, poor judgment, emotions, or external events.

*If I could start to draw on this kind of strength, I could begin to create the kind of life I can only dream about.*

You're right. However Quiet Time's benefits don't end there! Consider this. Imagine quieting your mind as a way to relax deeply. Do you even know how it feels to be mentally serene?

*Would this be how I felt as a child when I used to lie on my back watching the cloud formations in the sky? Or when I was completely enthralled by a bug crawling over the dew drops on a leaf? I could just be there, existing, carefree, fully immersed for hours in something seemingly important only to me.*

When we were children, we had all the time in the world to be free in our minds. Unfortunately, most of us started getting conflicting and hard-driving messages:

grow up, quit daydreaming, do what you are told, be productive, consider others, it's not good to waste time, you can relax when you're finished your work.

Free time is not a lazy childish preoccupation or a selfish desire that we must sacrifice so that we can take on our real adult responsibilities. Every day throughout our lives, we need to take time out.

Quieting our minds is a valuable means of releasing tension. Tension causes all kinds of problems if it builds up in our bodies. Often we turn to some inappropriate tension-release like food when we are desperate to free ourselves from our frenzied, hurried, or stressful state. Food can be a crutch that works to numb the brain by temporarily easing that tension, but in the long run, eating for the wrong reasons only creates more problems.

Alternately, people turn away from food when they are stressed. The more pressured they feel in their lives, the more rigid they become in their thinking and eating. They shift their focus to what they know and do well. This gives them a false sense of control, although here too, while the restricting may seem to ease their minds, it becomes a problem in itself, rather than a solution.

When you know how to quiet your mind, you can take time out throughout your day to pause and release built-up tension. This is what you need—a powerful and natural stress management tool that will help you reduce your risk of developing all kinds of stress-related symptoms.

*I thought that anxiety was a natural state to be in. I can always find something to feel anxious about.*

Hurrying, worrying, and feeling anxious are just bad habits, not expressions of your true nature. Your true nature is one of inner harmony and peace.

This doesn't mean that you can look forward to a state of constant bliss or euphoria. You will still experience your full range of emotions from the most painful to the most joyous. The difference is that any negative emotions you experience will be temporary. Anger, fear, sadness, confusion, doubt, anxiety, helplessness, frustration, apathy, or loneliness will dissolve into a more expansive base of positive emotion which is your true nature. You are meant to be sustained by emotions such as love, peace, patience, trust, security, appreciation, aliveness, forgiveness, and integrity. You will always come back to this fundamental state as long as you take the time every day to nurture that level.

*Do you have any suggestions to make this easy for me?*
*Would watching T.V. or reading count for Quiet Time?*

When you are watching television or reading (even a self-help book), your mind is still actively engaged in something outside yourself. While reading can be informative and relaxing, eventually you need to set even this aside, so that you can be with yourself directly. Take one more bold step on your behalf. Trust that your greatest source of wisdom is inside you and not in any external source, no matter how worthwhile and respected these other sources may be.

Even activities like physical exercise, walking, gardening, and other relaxing hobbies don't count as Quiet Time if your mind is still active. You won't benefit at all if you are busy worrying, analyzing your progress, putting yourself down, comparing yourself to others, planning meals, calculating the calories you're burning, or fantasizing.

There are some acceptable variations of the basic Quiet Time technique with which you may initially feel more comfortable. These measures can ease the transition from nonstop mental activity to a state of inner calmness.

Consider taking a bubblebath. Light a candle. Turn on some soft romantic, classical, or new-age music. Put some logs on the fire. Sink into your favorite easy chair.

Look out your window and watch the rain. Spend time outdoors, immersing yourself in nature. Watch the leaves, a waterfall, a sunset, some birds or squirrels. Take a long stroll or bike ride. Walk your dog.

Turn to philosophical readings. There are some wonderful sources of insight and inspiration in the written word. Embrace them! Let them touch your soul. Realize that you want to get beyond the words. First, read a brief selection to capture its essence. Then let go of the words, staying with the warm feelings that they evoke in you. To fully benefit, you need those accompanying moments of silent reflection.

Write in your journal whatever thoughts come to you. Then, sit for a while just to open up to your intuitive wisdom. Sometimes, in our determination to find immediate answers, we work too hard trying to solve life's problems intellectually. Rather than allow ourselves to live in the question, we push to find the answer. We leave little room for true insight and creative solutions.

Listen to relaxation or meditation tapes. Try some deep breathing exercises. Find out how to use simple concentration techniques. For example, consider closing your eyes and focusing on your natural breathing pattern without trying to alter it. Do this either by (1) concentrating on the tip of your nose or (2) repeating cycles of counting backward from ten to one to the rhythm of your breathing. Allow yourself five or ten minutes to do this.

Take up *Tai Chi* or yoga, but be patient with yourself. You can't learn either discipline in ten easy lessons. Become more sensitive to how your body feels as it moves in space, as you walk, run, stretch, dance, or swim. Consider getting a massage, facial, or pedicure. Draw. Paint. Play the piano.

Let yourself play. True play isn't tainted by aggressive competition, dead seriousness, self-consciousness, or guilt for taking time out. Instead, it has the qualities of being engaging, lighthearted, considerate of others, personally challenging and, of course, pure fun!

Be committed to bringing an increased awareness or mindfulness to any activity you are engaged in, be it ironing, baking, gardening, being with your children, or lovemaking. In essence, you are cultivating a presence—bringing a new richness to these experiences rather than being on automatic pilot, splitting your attention, or drifting off in unrelated thought.

Contemplation or prayer can be calming and healing. It can be a time for you to be in the presence of God, a time to honor the spiritual level in you. Here too, inner silence, receptivity and openness are important. Your prayers will not count as Quiet Time if you are busy chatting it up or asking for favors.

Meditation is another form of Quiet Time, but it is not necessary to use formal meditation. Many people prefer a less structured approach, one that is more natural or suited to their personal lifestyles. As long as you have found an approach to quieting your mind that works for you and feels right, trust that you can discover what is best for you. Above all, know that you can keep it simple.

This reminds me of a lesson that a dear friend of mine learned a long and laborious way. Pam came to me about ten years ago struggling with a food problem and severe depression. Even though she was logically inclined and intellectually brilliant, she was fascinated by our discussions of Quiet Time and meditation. Pam was, and still is, a medical researcher by profession. In her determination to find the best way to meditate, she turned Quiet Time into a major personal research project. She spent countless hours intensely pouring over journal publications and books—anything she could get her hands on—as well as committing herself to meditation practices and workshops.

On occasion, I would suggest to her that she might be going overboard in her search. However, Pam did not know how to keep things simple—she didn't believe in uncomplicated answers. She had her own plan in place and had to find out what she needed in her own way.

In the years that followed, Pam came to some interesting conclusions. One day she called me to say, "I have finally discovered that the best way for me to take Quiet Time is to sit down in the morning with a cup of coffee." In other words, she did not need any elaborate instructions, guided imagery tapes, special yoga positions, mantras, meditation retreats, or extensive scientific research. She simply needed to sit down with her self and truly experience the silence.

Regardless of the strategies that you learn to create a state of inner calm, you want to reach the point where you can sit with a quiet mind and do nothing else. Realize that, even then, thoughts will come to you—you can't turn off all thoughts—but they will be of a different quality. They're not part of your usual active thinking routine. Instead, they emerge from an inner source because you have created some space in your mind for them. This complementary form of thinking relates to insight, inspiration, and healing. It is reflective thought. As you learn to listen to the silence, you will begin to hear your inner voice.

The more you build Quiet Time into your daily life, the more you will begin to use it as a tool to help you. I recall one client who remarked that for many years she was looking for a magic pill to solve all her problems. When she came to my workshop, she soon realized that there was no magic pill and that she had to do all the work. Interestingly, the more she experienced the multifaceted, nourishing nature of Quiet Time, the more she realized that it was her magic pill. She now knows that she needs Quiet Time in her life every day for many different reasons. And she makes sure that she takes it!

## Gaining Inner Strength

*I guess for so long I have been hoping someone or something would save me. I now see I have to save myself.*

You don't need someone else to save you. When you take responsibility for yourself, something quite special happens. You connect with a remarkably empowering process. You can outgrow problems that may have otherwise destroyed you.

In her book *The Aquarian Conspiracy*, Marilyn Ferguson describes the work of Swiss psychoanalyst Carl Jung who captured the essence of this transformational process decades ago:

*"Some higher or wider interest arose on the person's horizon, and through this widening of*

*his view the problem lost its urgency. It was not solved logically in its own terms but faded out in contrast to a new and stronger life-tendency. It was not repressed and made unconscious but merely appeared in a different light."*

In your case, the insoluble problem is your problem with food. The higher or wider interest relates to an intense need to connect with your true self and a new love and appreciation for life. In a way that will be amazing to you, your crazy eating will start to lose hold of you as you grow stronger in yourself.

*I have heard of people who have come through against all odds. They refuse to give up. They triumph, rising above their difficulties. Whether they suffer from ill health or struggle with some other seemingly-insurmountable personal circumstances, they find within themselves the reason and strength to remain optimistic. I want to be one of those people.*

You have what you need to heal yourself. Remember, everyone has these innate abilities, although few use them. No matter how weak you feel, your inner self is wise and strong. When you are silent, you can listen to it and draw from its strength.

When you connect with your inner self, you will find that you can let go of your food and body focus. The diet mentality and body-oriented view of yourself will appear superficial and unappealing. You will know that life has profound significance far beyond how you look, what you wear, what you do, what you have, and who you know. This realization will surface intuitively. Once experienced, it is never lost or forgotten.

Deep down, you want to take care of yourself, and you want to evolve. As you listen to your inner voice, you will find it increasingly more difficult to follow a life-path that is not good for you. You will no longer tolerate unhealthy, self-defeating patterns of thinking. You will no longer allow yourself to neglect your body. You will strive for more balance and integration in all facets of your life.

Let's go back one more time to the people I introduced earlier. Some of them can relate to this healing experience. Determined to get to the root of their problems with food and eating, they confronted themselves. They opened their minds. They took responsibility. They let themselves learn in the true sense of the word. They discovered an inner stronghold that fostered resourcefulness and resilience in the face of setbacks and obstacles. Their life goals became motivated by intrinsic values and needs. These individuals now share the uplifting beliefs of our *fifth category*.

Pat is a testimonial to the power of transformation. For so long, he feigned innocence, choosing to blame others for his compulsive eating and unhappiness. One day he decided he was sick of playing victim; he could no longer fool or abandon himself. Rather than numb himself with food, he started facing his painful and frightening emotions, while at the same time, letting himself experience feelings like appreciation and love. Rather than hide behind his weight, Pat took his place in the world as a sensitive, worthwhile, capable, attractive man. Rather than ignore his inner self, he claimed it and developed a profound spiritual sense. This spiritual dimension sustained him and allowed him to be optimistic through some trying and turbulent times. Once he took full responsibility, both his eating and his weight began to stabilize.

Through therapy, Cheryl found that her unhealthy patterns extended beyond crazy eating to include compulsive spending, promiscuity, and egotistical self-absorption. Although she was not particularly eager to acknowledge these traits, she recognized them as signals that she must work on herself. She began to acknowledge her deep-seated negativity, fears, and insecurities. She found the courage to let go of her perfect image so that she could explore what was underneath. Initially, she feared that she might exacerbate her problems by taking that leap, but she knew that she had no choice but to face the unknown and to find a new life-path. When Cheryl quieted her mind, she felt something stirring—a spiritual awareness she could depend on to guide her. As her wisdom and sense of responsibility grew, she found she had no use for crazy eating or any other obsessions. When Cheryl reassessed her progress a year later, she was amazed. Even she found it hard to believe a person could change so much.

A young woman with a traumatic past, Sandy has made the important realization that at her core she cannot be touched by life events. Since gleaning this insight through counseling, she is starting to heal herself. As her inner resources grow, Sandy is beginning to trust that she can resolve some disturbing issues related to being physically, emotionally, and sexually abused when she was young. She is beginning to appreciate a longtime supportive and loving husband. She is regaining a sense of enjoyment in daily living. She is taking pride in her newly-developing coping abilities, aware that she is dealing well with a complicated life. No longer willing to jeopardize her physical health, Sandy is determined to nourish her body. While there are still ups and downs with food, they are becoming less frequent and severe. Sandy feels a warm glow inside. She knows that she has the resources to lead a full life.

*These stories are inspiring! There's something solid and real about this. I know that this is how I want to be.*

Then give yourself permission to explore who you are—freely, openly, and fully. Acknowledge your intrinsic hunger to lead a meaningful life, for that's when miracles happen. Old battles dissolve. Your task is not to manipulate, substitute, or reform your behaviors, but to transform or heal yourself.

*What exactly is a transformation?*

Transformation can be defined as a restructuring, a rebirth, an awakening. Psychosynthesist Anne Yeomans sees it as "the falling apart of old known ways of being and the coming together...of new more evolved ways of being."

I intentionally use the words *transformation* and healing, rather than *cure, recovery,* or *normalization* to describe this kind of self-change process. When you transform or heal yourself, you connect with your inner or spiritual self. You naturally transcend the narrow boundaries by which you have lived. You let go of your destructive patterns as you evolve because they no longer fit.

The image that comes to mind when I think of the process of transformation is that of a caterpillar turning into a butterfly. Just as the butterfly can't go back to the caterpillar stage, you can't step back into a less-evolved form of yourself. Instead, you move into a more mature stage, taking with you what is essential and shedding what you no longer need.

*While this all sounds inviting, I have a lingering fear. Don't you think that if I take this route, it may lead me*

*to become self-centered? I know I want to change, but it is not so simple. I have other people to think about.*

Yes, you have responsibilities to others, but you also have responsibilities to yourself. I call this a self-caring route, rather than a selfish one. As long as you consider others, you are entitled to live your life in a way that works for you. Genuine love and respect for others are natural outgrowths of true self-caring. Personal growth is not about being insensitive, hurtful, arrogant, self-righteous, neglectful, deceitful, or self-centered.

Trust that you will have even more to offer others if you take care of yourself. If you don't take full responsibility for yourself, you will suffer the consequences. No one else can do your inner work for you.

*I used to sense that there was more that I needed to learn about myself. But the opportunity never arose, so I concluded early in life that it was foolish to think there was more to my inner nature. Now you are saying my inner self is real, and that it is a central consideration in getting well. That is not a common point of view—not in the media, in schools, or among health professionals. How do I discover who I am and keep it alive for myself, especially when no one seems to support me or give me the chance?*

You have asked a perceptive and loaded question—one that brings the underlying source of your eating difficulties into sharp focus.

## Conditioning

We all learn our beliefs, values, and behaviors in the process of growing up. Because we were dependent on others in our formative years, we learned to look outside ourselves for cues about what we needed and what was real. For many of us, that meant learning patterns of relating to the external, tangible world, but not to our inner, experiential world. In effect, we closed the door on our selves.

By the time we reached adulthood, many of us long since ceased to believe that we had any innate worth or wisdom. No one helped us to understand that we're spiritual beings! Instead, we were molded by others' interpretations of what is acceptable, appropriate, desirable, important, and real.

Be it family, friends, the school system, the media, religion, the business world, or our own misguided notions—outside sources have shaped our identities and continue to do so. Many of us live with these false perceptions of ourselves for our entire lives.

That is what is so insidious about conditioning. It's so subtle that often we do not realize what is happening even after we begin to suffer the consequences. We would like to believe that we have escaped the tyranny of conditioning, but few of us truly have.

If our early years were particularly traumatic and our environments injurious, we may have drawn especially damaging conclusions about ourselves and our world. We may have resorted to extreme measures to cope with these overwhelming experiences. As a way to survive in a tough, dangerous, unfair, crazy, hurtful, or unpredictable world, many of us buried ourselves under layers and layers of elaborate defenses, distorted perceptions, and unresolved hurts.

In trying to hide from life's pains and injustices, we even hide from ourselves. Sadly, when it is finally safe to surface, we are lost inside. We do not realize that we have the resources within to live differently, and we are afraid of the unknown.

*Does it always go back to our families? Did we all start to get off track as children?*

It does not help to focus on one simple cause. Even when our families have been sources of loving attention and counsel, we can still get off track. We all move beyond our home environments into a society where we can fall victim to other influences.

Many well-known authors have examined what happens to us in the shaping process. In *Young Man Luther,* Erik Erikson states, "The most deadly of all sins is the mutilation of a child's spirit." The American psychiatrist Eric Fromm says, "The pity in life today is that most of us die before we are fully born." The American educator Leo Buscaglia comments, "We are so ruled by what people tell us we must be that we have forgotten who we are."

There is a poem by an unknown author that I find particularly touching. To me, this poem says it all.

### *About School*

*He always wanted to say things. But no one understood.*

*He always wanted to explain things. But no one cared.*

*So he drew.*

*Sometimes he would just draw and it wasn't anything. He wanted to carve it in stone or write it in the sky.*

---  ❧·❧·❧  ---

*He would lie out on the grass and look up in the sky and it would be only him and the sky and the things inside that needed saying.*

*And it was after that, that he drew the picture. It was a beautiful picture. He kept it under the pillow and would let no one see it.*

*And he would look at it every night and think about it. And when it was dark, and his eyes were closed, he could still see it.*

*And it was all of him. And he loved it.*

*When he started school he brought it with him. Not to show anyone, but just to have it with him like a friend.*

*It was funny about school.*

*He sat in a square, brown desk like all the other square, brown desks and he thought it should be red.*

*And his room was a square, brown room. Like all the other rooms. And it was tight and close. And stiff.*

*He hated to hold the pencil and the chalk, with his arm stiff and his feet flat on the floor, stiff, with the teacher watching and watching.*

*And then he had to write numbers. And they*

*weren't anything. They were worse than the letters that could be something if you put them together.*

*And the numbers were tight and square and he hated the whole thing.*

*The teacher came and spoke to him. She told him to wear a tie like all the other boys. He said he didn't like them and she said it didn't matter.*

*After that they drew. And he drew all yellow and it was the way he felt about morning. And it was beautiful.*

*The teacher came and smiled at him. "What's this?" she said. "Why don't you draw something like Ken's drawing? Isn't that beautiful?"*

*It was all questions.*

*After that his mother bought him a tie and he always drew airplanes and rocket ships like everyone else. And he threw the old picture away.*

*And when he lay out alone looking at the sky, it was big and blue and all of everything, but he wasn't anymore.*

*He was square inside and brown, and his hands were stiff, and he was like anyone else. And the thing inside him that needed saying didn't need saying anymore.*

*It had stopped pushing. It was crushed. Stiff.*

*Like everything else.*

The poem, *About School*, identifies the profound issues that affect someone with an eating problem, such as the devastating effects of being molded by external forces, losing touch with one's inner voice, and in time resigning oneself to a life without intrinsic meaning.

The silencing of one's inner voice through conditioning is not a rare occurrence. It happens every time:

- a woman looks into a mirror and berates herself because she is a size twelve instead of a size eight.

- someone measures out precisely three ounces of chicken, hoping to be satisfied with a mini-salad with low calorie dressing for dinner, and reluctantly puts the bread away because it is not allowed in Week One of the latest diet plan.

- someone flips through the page of a glossy magazine only to feel inferior because his/her own attributes or possessions do not match the impeccable airbrushed images there.

- the fashion section in a newspaper applauds the latest trend: a creation that could only look good on a five-foot eleven reed-thin mannequin.

- someone falls victim to opportunists who promise financial and career success, instant beauty, irresistible sex appeal, or easy enlightenment.

- someone is offered a quick chemical cure for depression, anxiety, insomnia, or binge eating, with no mention of alternatives that might provide more rewarding forms of self-care and self-responsibility.

- an offhand, selfish, or cruel comment burrows its way into a person's heart as if it were an eternal truth.

- a young child witnesses another bitter dispute between his parents and stores away in his memory bank the harsh words and physical violence, accepting that it is normal.

- a child tunes out in her mind as an intrusive hand fondles her body.

- a coach chastises the members of his prized athletic team, claiming that their performance is weak because they are fat.

- well-meaning individuals take their efforts to reach that pinnacle of perfection just a little too far, only to destroy themselves.

---- ❦❦❦ ----

When we are continuously misguided, degraded, violated, ignored, or coerced, the light within us can dim. It can even seem to go out. It's as if our essence or life force is extinguished, with no hope of being rekindled or regenerated.

Yet, the flame of the inner self can't be extinguished, no matter how lost we get or how bleak and desperate our lives become. Just as the smallest candle burns bright even in the darkest night, so the inner self will survive all despair. It is there for us to claim as our own.

### Opening to a Deeper Level

*I want this goodness you are talking about.*

Then let yourself be open to it!

Family psychotherapist Virginia Satir has said, "We are all cosmic jokes and sacred beings." Without a healthy perspective, we can't understand and accept our dark side for what it is. Instead, we get trapped in it by condemning ourselves. We don't see our sacredness.

It is time that you start to see your difficulties in a more appropriate context. You developed problems with food not because you are inherently weak, unworthy, or unlucky, but because you strayed too far from who you are.

*If my behavior is a loud and clear sign that I'm neglecting my true self, what happens when people don't get a sign like mine? Does it mean that their lives are on track?*

Many people appear to be well-balanced, but if they are not sensitive to this inner level, in truth, they do not know who they are. They still have some important learning to do although they may not realize it.

Paradoxically, it is often through hardship, when old ways don't work and our resources seem to fail us, that we stop to take stock of our situations. Sometimes it is only as a last-ditch effort to help ourselves that we let ourselves embark on an inward journey. Much to our amazement, that is when we encounter a self that is far more beautiful than we could have ever imagined.

The irony of how we find what we are looking for when and where we least expect it reminds me of the story of the man who wanders the world in search of the most precious jewel. When he becomes exhausted by his explorations, he returns to the place where he started only to find the jewel on his forehead.

*How does life become different when we awaken to this deeper level?*

Those who connect with this way of living have a gentle, humane life philosophy. Their way has not given them less; it has brought them more. They are healthy-minded individuals and free thinkers. They have peace of mind and a center from which to deal with the world. They feel connected with their potential. They live and love life deeply and have a true conscience.

They resist conformity, preferring to carve out rich, individualistic lives. They focus on quality rather than quantity and stay true to their values despite what others do. They have compassion and seek to lessen human suffering. They wish for others what they want for themselves. Their most profound experiences could be considered mystical or spiritual. They value solitude.

That does not mean these people are perfect or that they have perfect lives. Rather, they have developed more of who they truly are. Consequently, they experience life more fully and confront all challenges more effectively.

They are aware that they have imperfections and issues to work on. They know how to learn in a way that allows them to grow. They continue to address real issues, refine their personalities, and strive to actualize their potential. They have the necessary insight and strength to do so, and they know they can't settle for less.

Humanistic psychologist Abraham Maslow described individuals with these kinds of characteristics as *self-actualized*. Some experts scoff at the notion of self-actualization or self-realization, claiming it is idealistic to think that we can live according to some kind of higher, never-mind spiritual, nature.

Yet, there are people who are deeply aware and leading inspired lives. Often, their truths appear simplistic to those of us who value our complex, analytical minds, when ironically, it is our cluttered thinking and intellectualization that keep us from experiencing this incredible richness for ourselves.

*The spiritual level is so valuable. Why doesn't everyone wake up?*

There are too many people who believe that there is no spiritual self or that it is impossible to find it outside the context of a narrow religious path. Others mistakenly believe that they are already awake or fully conscious just because they are exploring an internal realm of themselves or have an intellectual understanding of what self may be. In general, our society belittles the spirit. Science dismisses it. Religion often distorts or complicates it.

Elizabeth Kubler-Ross, the American psychiatrist who has studied death and dying and paradoxically life and living, states this: "...our concern must be to *live* while we're alive—to release our inner selves from the spiritual death that comes with living behind a facade designed to conform to external definitions of who and what we are." Her message serves as a challenge for every human being who wishes to lead a full life.

*What will guide me on my journey to my self?*

Inner work is meant to be basic. While it is not my place to put you on a specific path—you need to find your own—I suggest that you keep things simple. Remember, you want to get in touch with what is already inside you. Everything important comes back to a few fundamental ideas. You need to be patient while you work and rework these ideas until they start to show results for you.

Do not look for easy answers or external solutions. No amount of reading, studying, attending workshops or support groups, or exploring new-age paraphernalia will substitute for quieting your mind and looking within. Furthermore, no amount of quieting your mind and looking within will help you to get well unless you are also prepared to face your issues and to take full responsibility for your life. You are meant to learn certain life-lessons. You can begin when you are ready to make the genuine commitment to your personal and spiritual growth.

*This gives me so many new options.*

If you can look at your problem with food in a broader context, it will begin to make sense. Then you can focus your attention on issues that are truly relevant. The essential questions no longer are "How do I sort out my eating?" and "Why am I so useless or weak?" Instead, they are "How do I learn from this darkness and pain?" and "How do I nurture myself?"

You are meant to be whole—integrated in body, mind, and spirit. When you live your life in a way that fits, you no longer feel as if you are lost in a vast ocean or swimming against the current. You live in the natural flow of life.

*I have always wanted to believe that my life had significance. I am beginning to regain the hope that I lost somewhere along the way.*

It is time for you to re-establish that genuine belief in your self and a higher spiritual order. You can create a context for optimal growth.

If you are intent on helping yourself, be open to all of your healing options. Look carefully, deliberately, and without apology at alternative ways of helping yourself. Make a commitment to work on that inner level, to nourish your self. Only you can activate your inner healing capacity, the most powerful healing force of all.

Wherever you find people who value greater truths and goodness, you will find individuals who can help you to foster your healing potential. You may be fortunate enough to have a doctor, therapist, minister, or teacher who already lives by such a life-view or philosophy. You may find support among family members and friends. You may be inspired by words of wisdom from authors or speakers. Others in your situation can provide understanding and support if they, too, are looking for meaning in life.

As you continue on your healing journey, you will sense that even greater potential is being unleashed. That is when the higher purpose of your eating problem will present itself to you. You will find that your suffering and learning have been more instructive than you ever imagined. Listen closely to your inner voice; opportunities to take your true place in the world will arise.

I know that you are meant to make a unique contribution to humanity. It is up to you to find this purpose. Open your eyes and you will see disparity, strife, imbalance, ignorance, and the need for healing almost everywhere. Individually, we need to heal ourselves. Collectively, we can begin to heal our world. You can't assume your larger responsibility if you don't know who you are, if you center your life on issues of body and food.

*How is it that you seem to know where I am and where I need to be?*

I know where you are because I was there about fifteen years ago. I, too, had a severe eating disorder. I once saw life in a distorted, limiting way and experienced my life as hell. I now live each day fully because I have taken responsibility for myself.

If I had not gone through the healing process myself, I could not speak with the confidence that I do. I know where you are. I know that you have boundless potential. I know the process you need to connect with to transform.

*So what is my next step?*

First I would like to point out that you have already taken some important steps, whether you realize it or not. You have opened your mind significantly. You are more patient and honest. You are facing your situation directly. You know how you want to live. You are willing to learn. These qualities will serve you well as you proceed.

This conversation can mark a new beginning for you. Let this be the occasion when you made the decision to expand your vision to include the inner realm. In her powerfully transforming book *The Aquarian Conspiracy,* Marilyn Ferguson reminds us that we have every reason to believe in our potential to help ourselves and tells us why this is so:

> *"Something in us is wiser and better informed than our ordinary consciousness. With such an ally within us, why should we do it alone?"*

In her beautiful book *The Unfolding Self,* another visionary, Molly Brown, urges us to wholeheartedly embrace our unfolding destinies:

*"We must accept and develop our vast, unexpressed potential, individually and together. We must transform the patterns of fear and doubt which hold us back from being all we can be for ourselves and for the world. The task of transformation begins within the heart and mind of each one of us."*

If you wish, we can meet again to explore the transformational process in greater depth, in carefully-guided steps. Meanwhile, now that you have opened your mind, I ask you to open your heart.

Healing yourself from an eating problem is not about desperately seeking external or surface solutions. It is about listening to what is already inside you.

Your spiritual self is there now, waiting to gently guide you, to heal you, and to help you to realize your unique life purpose.

*I have learned a lot. You can count on me to come back.*

Know that you are welcome here any time.

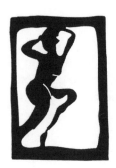

*The fundamental task which gives the key to many realizations is the silence of the mind . . . All kinds of discoveries are made, in truth, when the mental machinery stops, and the first is that if the power to think is a remarkable gift, the power not to think is even more so.*

- *Sri Aurobindo*

# Quiet Time

Quiet Time is time that we take to be with ourselves in inner silence. When we quiet our minds or suspend our logic, we allow for a quality of thinking that helps us to access our deeper being—our spirit. In this way, Quiet Time awakens us to our true natures and frees the process of spiritual growth. For centuries, philosophers, spiritual teachers, and visionaries have told us: solitude is the richness of self; give attention to the soul; lift the veil that separates you from your universal wisdom; and find a place of stillness so that heavenly forces can pour through you, recreate you, and use you for the betterment of humankind.

In time, if we are committed to the daily practice of Quiet Time, we experience its transforming effect. Our awareness opens. We allow ourselves to be inwardly guided. We know who we are and bring into our lives a richness of self that naturally alters our perceptions and values. We begin to follow through in ways that confirm that we know how to be true to ourselves, that life has meaning, and that we can help to enhance life for everyone. Unhealthy patterns of thought and behavior begin to dissipate. They no longer fit and never will.

While this inner process is best guided by an experienced teacher, you can begin by yourself by setting aside some time each day to practice. What follows is a simple description of Quiet Time.

## How to Take Quiet Time

- You cannot expect to quiet your mind in the midst of your normal daily activities, not when you are first learning how to do this. Set aside a block of time, at least fifteen minutes every day, to be with yourself in inner silence.

- Remember, this time is just for you. Put aside your worries, responsibilities, roles—everything that would distract you—no matter how important these concerns are during the rest of the day. Every day you need time away from your usual activities. You need a mental break.

- Do not wait too late to take Quiet Time. Learning how to quiet your mind requires considerable mental energy. If you are tired, you will not have the strength to practice or you may fall asleep.

- Give yourself permission to take this time. You want to take it without feeling guilty. Your daily life may be complex and filled to the brim with never-ending pressures, complications, and responsibilities, but the world will not fall apart if you set aside fifteen minutes at some time in your day. Even if you do not feel you deserve time out, it is what you need if you want to get well and to stay well. Think of it as an investment in yourself. It is time well spent, as you will soon discover.

- Choose a setting that is free from distractions—quiet, comfortable, not too hot, not too cold. Sit comfortably with your back straight. Do not lie down. Closing your eyes may help you to cut out external distractions, but do not get so relaxed that you fall asleep!

- As you begin Quiet Time, take a few deep breaths to center yourself. Remind yourself how important this time is for you, and open your mind to experience your self deeply. Slowly breathe in and out, in and out, in and out.

- Bring your attention to your thinking. You want to observe your thoughts with the intention of letting them go. So, for example, if a thought comes to mind related to an unfinished task, acknowledge it and gently usher it out of your mind with the reminder: "This may be important, but I will come back to it after Quiet Time. Right now, I just want to calm my mind." When another thought comes to mind, repeat the letting-go technique.

- The goal of Quiet Time is to calm and relax your mind and to suspend active thinking. This will allow you to access a more subtle, intuitive level of thought. This is how healing begins.

- Persevere. While you will experience considerable difficulties in your early attempts to still your mind, continue your daily practice. In time, your mind will start to co-operate; it will slow down. With daily practice, Quiet Time will become easier.

- Be eager and ready for insights and for positive change, but do not set deadlines or unrealistic expectations. Quiet Time has a pace of its own. It is not something that you can rush or force. Even if you do not see changes as soon as you might like, continue your daily practice. Important benefits occur before you can notice them. Given time, the benefits that come with mind-training, deep relaxation, reflection, and sensitivity to inner self and inner resources will be open to you.

- As your experience deepens, you will intuitively know the kind of Quiet Time that you need. There will be occasions when all that you want to do is to relax. At other times, you may wish to reflect on a personal issue to increase your understanding of it, or you may sense a need to sit with painful emotions and to work them through. You may want to use the time to evoke and develop inner qualities such as appreciation or patience. Or you may simply want to be mindful, giving your full attention to experiencing the present moment.

- With daily practice, Quiet Time will become much easier, even natural to you. You will find that you can slip into a reflective state without effort, whenever you want and wherever you are. You will know intuitively which kind of thinking process—active or reflective—is most suitable for every situation.

- Be committed to building Quiet Time into your everyday life. Quiet Time is a human need as essential as sleep. Nothing else can substitute for it. You need time out each day to be with yourself in inner silence. Consider this as your way of establishing and maintaining a meaningful relationship with your spiritual self.

# About the Author

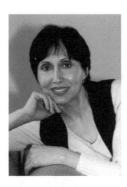

For fifteen years, Viola Fodor experienced the full range of eating disorders—binge eating, anorexia, and bulimia. Desperate to understand her problem and to help herself, she studied psychology and nutrition at university for seven of those years. Her self-help efforts were futile. Her problem worsened.

Then in 1981, Viola healed herself from her eating disorder by turning inward and allowing her deepest wisdom to guide her. She emerged from her despair with profound insight into the self-healing process and a powerful message to share with others. She was sure that she had tapped into some fundamental truths about well-being and personal transformation that would benefit countless others. In the same year, she established her private practice to help people who were struggling with similar disorders.

In *Desperately Seeking Self,* Viola draws from her own personal and professional experiences to bring a unique learning opportunity to readers. She extends a thoughtful, inspiring message to people who yearn to lead fulfilling lives but do not know how to proceed in the personal growth process.

Viola lives in Campbellville, Ontario. She counsels individuals with a full range of lifestyle concerns and leads workshops for professional and lay groups using a humanistic/transpersonal perspective.

If you would like more information on her programs and resource materials, you can write her in care of the Wellness Centre Inc., P. O. Box 364, Campbellville, Ontario, Canada L0P 1B0.

# About the Publisher

Since 1980, Gürze Books has specialized in providing quality information on eating disorders recovery, research, education, advocacy, and prevention. They also distribute *The Gürze Eating Disorders Bookshelf Catalogue,* which is used as a resource throughout the world.

# To Order

Copies of *Desperately Seeking Self* are available at bookstores and libraries or directly from Gürze Books.

## FREE Catalogue

The *Gürze Eating Disorders Bookshelf Catalogue* has more than 100 books and tapes on eating disorders and related topics, including body image, size-acceptance, self-esteem, feminist issues, and more. It is a valuable resource that is handed out by therapists, educators, and other health care professionals throughout the world.

**Gürze Books (PRK)**
**PO Box 2238**
**Carlsbad, CA 92018**
**(760) 434-7533**
**gzcatl@aol.com • www.gurze.com**